The Hay Fever Handbook

A progressive drug-free self-help programme which can give lasting relief from the torment of hay fever.

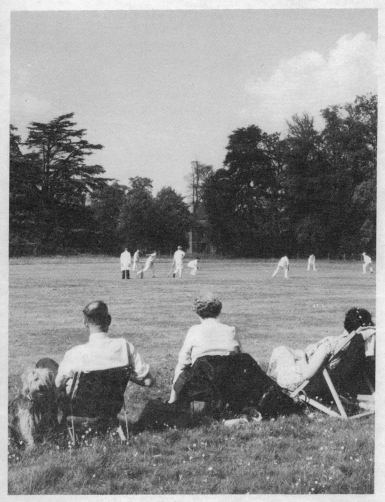

Pleasures lost . . .   (Photograph: Dennis Mansell)

The
Hay Fever
Handbook

A Summer Survival Plan

by

Roger Newman Turner
B.Ac., N.D., D.O., M.R.O.

THORSONS PUBLISHING GROUP

For Birgid
whose patience found
new reserves

First published 1988

British Library Cataloguing in Publication Data

Newman Turner, Roger
   The hay fever handbook: a summer survival
   plan.
   1. Hay-fever — Treatment   2. Self-care,
   Health
   I. Title
   616.2'02068   RC590

   ISBN 0-7225-1592-8

*Published by Thorsons Publishing Group,
Wellingborough, Northamptonshire,
NN8 2RQ, England.*

Printed in Great Britain by
Richard Clay Limited, Bungay, Suffolk

10 9 8 7 6 5 4

Contents

Acknowledgements

The preparation of a book exploring all forms of help for hay fever invariably entails drawing on the specialized knowledge of many people. My grateful thanks go to all those who gave generously of their time and expertise, and particularly to my colleagues Peter Goldman, Joseph Goodman and Martin Budd.

Otherwise the creation of *The Hay Fever Handbook* had strong shades of nepotism. Adam and Alison Newman Turner provided some of the recipes, as did my wife Birgid. Our son Julian Newman Turner did the graphics. They all earned my appreciation, not only for complying courteously with my requests.

Once again Lynne Metcalfe has laboured patiently through the task of transcribing my words on to screen and paper with a devotion that defies adequate gratitude.

Introduction

For hundreds of thousands of people the arrival of summer brings a time of torment and misery. The smarting eyes, streaming sinuses, and stuffy nose and head that herald the hay fever season often strike at the most inopportune times. It is an affliction which arrives at an early age and reaches its peak, for many sufferers, in their late teens, just when important exams are taking place. But it isn't just the young whose summers become a misery; increasing numbers of adults are reporting the onset of symptoms without any previous history of the problem.

Hay fever symptoms are caused by the body's reaction to the pollens from spring and summer plants. For this reason it is known in medical parlance as *pollinosis*, but there are similar symptoms which can be precipitated by other irritants, such as moulds and house-dust mites. These cause a condition known as *allergic rhinitis* which is virtually identical to hay fever.

Like the common cold, with which it is often confused, hay fever has made a great social impact on our lives, as indicated by the publication of the pollen count with the daily weather records throughout the summer. If the weather is bad you can always take an umbrella but the hay fever victim can only stay indoors or, perhaps, wear one of those goldfish bowl helmets!

In the midst of all this misery hay fever sufferers may feel pretty helpless but there are, in fact, many ways in which they can assist themselves. The latest knowledge about the role of nutrition and other physical measures to alleviate allergic disorders makes their prospects brighter than ever before. In this book I shall consider all the more effective treatments now available by which hay fever may not only be eased but eventually eradicated. Relief is possible without having to resort to the conventional drugs that make you feel dopey.

The age of allergy

We always like to have a scapegoat for our ailments. It used to be fashionable to blame 'a bug'. Now we live in the age of the allergy and when we feel unwell we say 'I must be allergic to something'. It is simply our way of shifting the responsibility for our health onto some outside agency instead of recognizing the self-healing and self-regulating capacity we all possess.

Hay fever is a typical allergy — rapid onset, severe discomfort, often no prior warning — but nature, usually considered the enemy, has provided many safe and effective resources for the relief of the hay fever sufferer. You no longer need to accept allergy as an inescapable burden you have to bear. It is not necessary to rely on drugs which confront the symptoms without correcting the cause. In this handbook I shall explain a wide range of easy to follow methods which have proved their worth for inumerable sufferers.

Simple herbal and homoeopathic remedies can be used for safe relief of the symptoms. New discoveries about food, as well as old and well-tried methods, are combined to bring you a selection of dietary approaches which can remove the basic causes of your allergy. Invigorating tonic measures can be undertaken using the resources available in your own home and The Hay Fever Reflex Workout is a simple massage routine, using special energy points, which you can do on yourself or your family. Altogether this handbook provides a programme for summer survival and effective year-round health care.

Does it really work?

All the recommendations I shall include in this book are safe natural procedures aimed at enhancing the body's own healing processes. They have all been found helpful by hay fever sufferers and have the added virtue of being harmless. In an age which has become accustomed to instant relief of symptoms by drugs (albeit with side-effects) people invariably expect immediate benefit from natural medicines and are inclined to give up if it isn't forthcoming. There is no wonder-cure for hay fever. The secret of success is patient application. Whilst many natural medicines can frequently be far more effective than drugs, and often quicker, a lasting improvement will take time.

There is still a need for much more research to be done on the methods described here but the most telling evidence is that thousands have been helped by their use. They are treatments, directed at your total health, which tackle the causes of hay fever and not merely the symptoms. The Fast Relief Plan, which is described in Chapter 16, is a revolutionary approach to hay fever, based on a number of the treatments explained in this book, which will bring speedy relief to most cases.

Positive action

So *now* is the time for action, not just on the one front but on several. Experience has shown that the best results are obtained by using a total health programme. Don't just wait for the hay fever season; start *now* to promote your all-round health and your body will take care of the symptoms. And in case you need professional guidance we shall consider the choices available to you from the leading complementary medicine systems.

Altogether there is a fascinating selection of supportive measures which you can use to survive the season of suffering. If they have helped somebody else with hay fever and are safe, I have tried to include them here because they may help you. But, above all, you will be able to help yourself to regain once more the real pleasures of summertime.

1 How Hay Fever Happens

The immune overkill

If you are among the millions who have to endure the misery of hay fever this may seem like a chapter of woe. When you've got hay fever it's pretty obvious and you don't much care how it happens as long as you can get rid of it. So, let me say straight away that this book will explain how you can do just that. Whatever the intricate mechanisms by which your body inflicts the symptoms on you, the management of hay fever depends on attention to your health as a whole and there are many ways in which you can do this to make your summers of discontent more glorious once again.

True hay fever is a seasonal illness which occurs when the body shows an exaggerated reaction to pollens and other fine particles in the atmosphere. The main symptoms are a prickly irritation of the nose and throat, leading to sneezing and a thin watery discharge, with itchiness and watering of the eyes. In more severe cases there may be swelling of the eyelids, even of the whole face, and there can be some breathing difficulty or wheeziness.

Is it really hay fever?

When hay fever first occurs it is often mistaken for a summer cold but these are usually confined to the nose and throat with thicker nasal catarrh. They may also be accompanied by the general aching of the limbs and swollen glands or headache which indicate the body's overall sense of crisis. With hay fever the crisis is very much more in the nose and eyes, with involvement of the chest in bad cases.

Hay fever is generally worst from May to September* when plants are most prolific with their pollens. It is an allergic reaction to the pollens but needs to be distinguished from similar symptoms caused by house dust or the spores from moulds and fungi which is a condition known as *allergic rhinitis*. Some people can also have similar symptoms due to excessive sensitivity without being allergic. This condition is *non-allergic rhinitis*. The management of all these disorders, and of the asthma which sometimes accompanies hay fever, is basically the same.

Most of us in normal health have a remarkable self-regulatory process which keeps our bodies in working order and protects them from undesirable intruders. Throughout the day and night we are exposed to a wide variety of chemical particles, bacteria, viruses, spores, and other organic matter, which might be a danger to us if they got into deeper tissues and organs.

Our defensive systems, however, learn to recognize what is foreign and reject or neutralize it. But for 10 per cent of the population these defensive mechanisms are a mixed blessing. It is estimated that over four million people in the United Kingdom suffer from hay fever with reactions to pollens from various trees, flowers, and grasses, and another two million have similar symptoms triggered by other particles causing rhinitis.

Whilst, for most of us, our bodies can keep pollens at bay without bothering us, the hay fever victim's body overreacts and releases excessive amounts of histamine, the substance which causes the itching, swelling, and watering of the eyes, nose, and throat.

The adaptation syndrome

The body responds to a crisis, be it an emotional shock or an unwelcome intruder in its tissues, by a sequence of events first described over forty years ago by Dr Hans Selye of Montreal, Canada. He called it the General Adaptation Syndrome.

According to Selye body defence mechanisms operate in three stages. The initial response to a foreign substance or micro-organism, or even a cut of the skin surface, is called the *alarm stage* during which scavenging cells and healing substances are released to clear up the area. Sometimes the activity is sufficient to generate some local heat giving rise to inflammation. When there is a more general reaction in the body there

* In the southern hemisphere the peak months are November to February

will be fever. Hay fever is not a real fever but it is so named because of the feverish symptoms which occur in reaction to grass pollens, especially at hay making time. The term is also applied to symptoms due to pollens which are released from many other plants at any time from April to September.

The second phase of the defensive mechanism is a *stage of resistance* when the body has successfully overcome the invader and maintains reasonable well-being in spite of its presence in the surroundings. Many people may have experienced a slightly prickly throat or eyes, with a runny nose, after their first exposure to a high concentration of pollen on a dry summer's day and then had no further trouble. Some years later, though, they may start getting symptoms again when the body defences have been worn down.

This is the *stage of exhaustion*. It sets in when the body can no longer sustain sufficient resistance because of constant exposure to the irritant and, more importantly, a gradual decline in its own functional ability. It is, therefore, important to consider how we can maintain healthy body defence to protect ourselves against hay fever and other allergies.

Who gets hay fever?

Hay fever is predominantly an affliction of the young, but can occur at any age. It generally starts in the 6-10 year olds and increases to over 10 per cent of the 10-15 year olds in the population. It may affect as many as 20 per cent of older children and students. It becomes a particular problem for students sitting important exams at the height of the season in June. They face either the torment of the streaming symptoms or the mind-dulling effect of many of the drugs used for their relief.

Plenty of adults also suffer from hay fever and a significant number of cases may not develop the condition until their thirties and forties or older. The onset of hay fever, in children or adults, may simply be the point of breakdown in the body's adaptive mechanisms. Children, however, have a much more vigorous immune system and are likely to have more acute, even feverish symptoms. Hay fever affects males more than females, but whether this is due to differences in the competence of the immune system between the sexes or simply to the fact that men are more commonly exposed to pollens is not clear.

Often the victim of hay fever is susceptible to other related conditions such as asthma and eczema. Hay fever patients have a two to three fold increased risk of developing asthma because of the nature of the mechanisms involved in the onset of the symptoms. They may be more inclined to have disorders which have an allergic basis, such as headaches, catarrh, and digestive troubles. The late onset hay fever person may have been subject to colds and catarrh or skin trouble in childhood which were suppressed by antibiotics, cold cures, and ointments.

As we explore the mechanisms of hay fever it will become apparent that it is not simply exposure to pollens which is responsible. The conditioning by our environment, eating habits, and hereditary tendencies all play a role, and the patterns of health and disease through our life have a common thread. Disease symptoms may have many manifestations but the underlying cause is basically a disharmony in bodily function.

Allergy

Our immune system protects us against foreign proteins by neutralizing them and mobilizing defence cells, but in some cases this activity can be too vigorous and causes unpleasant symptoms. People who react in this way are said to be *allergic*.

An allergy is an exaggerated self-damaging defence reaction to substances which are normally well tolerated. Most people get used to the many types of pollen which are in the air during the growing season of plants, but hay fever victims have an uncomfortable time because of their hypersensitivity to these minute particles. If their initial response is excessive they become sensitized to the triggering substance and each subsequent exposure causes an immediate or delayed reaction.

Substances which cause an allergic response, in this case pollens, are called *allergens*. Most allergens are protein particles which are not compatible with our own body proteins. They usually contain *antigens* which stimulate the formation of *antibodies* in the defensive system. Antibodies are specific to each type of foreign protein and always recognize them when they appear in the body again. During childhood many acute illnesses, such as measles, mumps, and chickenpox, stimulate antibodies which protect us for the rest of our lives. Breast milk also contains many substances essential to the development of a healthy immune system.

Immunoglobulins

The various types of antibodies are collectively known as *immunoglobulins*, some of which are formed only slowly, giving a delayed reaction as, for example, when some individuals react to a food like strawberries or shellfish which only cause trouble a day or two later. Immunoglobulin E (IgE), which is the main antibody involved in hay fever, causes an almost immediate reaction. Immunologists call this a Type 1 hypersensitivity. It commences a few minutes after exposure to the allergen, can be quite severe for 4-6 hours and then clears in 24 hours.

Lymphocytes

The cells which keep up the constant surveillance of our tissues are called the *lymphocytes*. They patrol the body in search of foreign particles and can normally distinguish them from those which are part of our own structure. Lymphocytes are produced mainly in the thymus, a mass of glandular tissue situated at the top of the chest, which is quite large and active in infants and children but gradually reduces to a small area of tissue in adults.

Lymphocytes produced by the thymus are known as T cells, of which there are two types, the T helper cells, which boost the immune system, and the T suppressor cells, which prevent it from going too far and destroying the body's own tissues.

Other lymphatic tissues also play an important role in our immune system, especially the appendix, tonsils, and glands of the neck, armpits, and groin. If any of these are removed early in life because they are enlarged or infected, such individuals are likely to develop more chronic disorders, including catarrh in sinuses and lungs, which increases the likelihood of hay fever as they get older.

Sensitization

The membranes lining the airways remove particles which become deposited on their surface by binding them in the protective mucous coat. The wave-like motion of the fine hair-like processes, the cilia, then move unwanted matter towards the pharynx, at the back of the mouth, from where it may be swallowed. The efficiency of this first line of defence depends on the quality of IgA.

If the membranes are weakened the pollen particles may penetrate to the underlying tissues where they induce a sequence of changes involving the lymphocytes, other scavengers, and the plasma cells to form IgE, the antibody which sensitizes the mast cells (figure 1). Mast cells are a large type of white blood cell, plentiful in the membranes of nose, sinuses, and lungs, which store several chemicals that may cause the symptoms of hay fever, the most common of which is histamine.

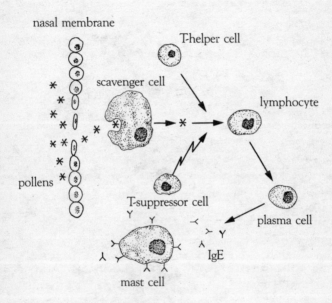

Figure 1. **The sequence of sensitization.**
Weak nasal membranes are penetrated by pollens which are engulfed by the scavenger cells. These pass the pollen molecules on to the lymphocytes which with the control of the T-cells, induce the production of antibody by the plasma cells. The antibody 'primes' the mast cell.

Histamine

Of all the symptoms triggered by allergic reactions the horrors of hay fever must rank as the highest. The immediate response to pollen of itching eyes, sneezes, and streaming nasal discharge is due mainly to histamine. Histamine is one of the chemicals which

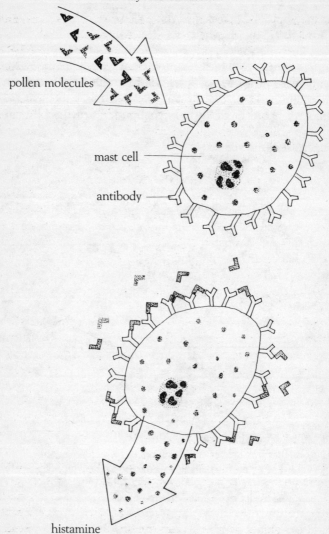

pollen molecules

mast cell

antibody

histamine

Figure 2. **Mast cell response.**
The molecules of antibody (IgE) on the mast cell are coded to recognize the pollen molecules which lock onto them and trigger the release by the cell of histamine.

maintains normal brain function but in excess quantity it contributes to depression and spells trouble for the allergic individual.

When further pollen molecules come in contact with the IgE on the surface of the sensitized mast cells their response is a release of histamine with other irritating chemicals.

Antihistamines are a popular form of symptomatic relief but they only improve matters by reducing the amount of histamine in the tissues. They don't reduce the sensitivity or its causes and they generally make the victim feel drowsy.

Testing for allergy

Not everyone who experiences unpleasant symptoms of the nose and throat is truly allergic. True allergy is a reaction to foreign protein molecules involving the immune system with the release of immunoglobulins. There can be many symptoms that are similar to hay fever in which immunoglobulins do not play a part. Non-allergic rhinitis, for example, is a condition in which the nasal membranes are irritated by various factors causing a constant runny nose.

A careful assessment of the problem by a doctor or naturopath will usually be sufficient to determine whether or not your symptoms are due to an allergic reaction. The type of reaction and its timing are good indications and the association of sneezes, itches, and wheezes, with the times of high pollen levels in the air is a fairly clear confirmation of hay fever. It is at either end of the summer when other spores and moulds may be involved that the identification of the allergen becomes more difficult. In severe cases it may help to identify the offending substances by special tests.

The *skin prick test* is the most common method of testing for allergies. A solution of the test substance is applied to a small area of the skin on the arm which has been scraped with a sterile needle or it is injected just beneath the surface. The appearance of a wheal or blister within 20 minutes signifies an allergic response to the substance tested. A number of different substances, or various types of pollens, can be tested at the same time. A variation on this test is to apply the test substance to the scratch with a plaster.

Although skin tests may help to identify specific pollens to which you may be sensitive, thus enabling you to steer clear of the offending plants in the future, they are not entirely reliable. Some substances may react at the skin and not internally, whilst others which cause symptoms may prove negative in the test. At least 5 per cent of symptom-free subjects have positive pollen skin tests.

Blood tests can be used to detect an allergic disposition but not so readily to identify the allergen. The blood can be tested for antibodies such as IgE, histamine levels, and immune complexes (the range of chemical substances released for its defence when the body is under threat). The Cytotoxic Test is a procedure in which changes in the blood cells are observed after they have been brought into contact with specific foods or other allergens. As with many allergy tests it is open to error.

Other tests of food sensitivity, such as the Sublingual Test (placing a few drops of a special preparation of the test food under the tongue), and Pulse Test (measuring pulse rate at intervals after eating specific foods to note any increase which would indicate sensitivity) are not relevant to your hay fever, except where unsuitable foods may be causing a breakdown of general body health and resistance, making your nasal membranes more vulnerable to penetration by the pollens.

There are a number of other ways of identifying specific pollen sensitivities which make use of the body's electromagnetic energy and these are explained in Chapter 13.

Although it can be helpful to know which substances trigger off your allergic response so that you may avoid close contact with them, you could end up a recluse as you develop more and more sensitivities if you do nothing about the basic causes of your allergy. It is far more important to know *why* you are allergic than to what you are allergic.

Pollens

Hay fever is the price its unfortunate victims pay for us all to enjoy the beauty of blossoms in the spring, or the undulations of a mature meadow in the summer breeze. As plants reach their maximum growth they try to ensure their survival by releasing millions of minute granules into the air. These are the pollen grains, some of which will find other plants of the same species to propagate seeds for the next season's growth.

Because of their important life-giving properties, pollen grains are rich in protein, but when they penetrate the membranes of the nose, sinuses, and lungs, they can set up an allergic reaction. Each type of pollen may contain a variety of different allergenic substances.

The most colourful flowers are designed to attract insects which then carry the pollen from plant to plant. It is the less showy plants whose pollens cause the most trouble. Their spores have to be finer so they can be carried by the wind and they are much more likely to trigger allergic responses since they are easily inhaled and can more readily penetrate the mucous membranes.

The grasses, certain trees without flowers, and plants such as Mugwort and Ragweed, are the most common sources of pollens. The vivid yellow patchwork of the countryside in the spring reflects the increasing agricultural production of oilseed rape which is another plant that triggers hay fever. Some of the trees release their pollens in April or May, which causes early snuffles and itches, but the worst time in the U.K. is June, just before and during the hay-making season. According to a survey of hay fever sufferers carried out by *Which?* magazine in 1985, only 9 per cent experienced trouble in April, whilst 77 per cent werre afflicted in the peak month of June. This is also the time, unfortunately, when many school-children and students are taking important exams.

In the U.S.A. ragweed is the principal pollen producer. One plant can release ten billion grains which can be spread over several miles on a breezy day. The insect pollinated plants, such as chrysanthemum, can only really cause sensitivity by direct contact.

Most people are allergic to specific pollens, but if you are hypersensitive you are likely to react to a wide range of them. Each type of pollen creates its own antibodies, however, and if you become allergic to grass pollen this may not necessarily make you react to that from trees. You can, though, get a cross reaction between pollens from different grasses, different trees, or different plants.

Pollen count

The concentration of pollen in the atmosphere may be of considerable interest to the hay fever sufferer, so much so that the figure is usually published in the newspapers along with the weather reports. The trouble is that it is not a forecast and only records the average level reached the day before, but it may explain why you felt so bad and suggest that you might have been wiser not to venture

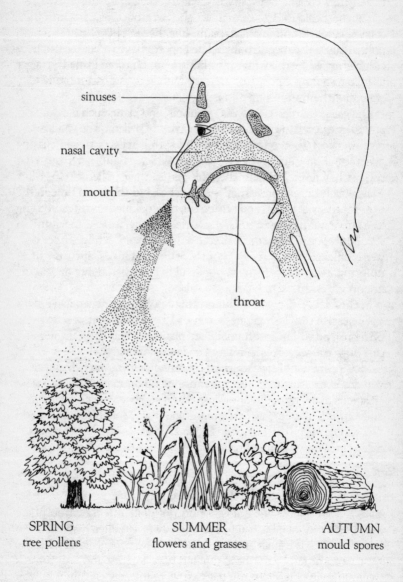

SPRING
tree pollens

SUMMER
flowers and grasses

AUTUMN
mould spores

Figure 3. Peak times for pollens and spores.

out! Yesterday's count, however, gives you a good idea of what to expect today if the weather isn't changing.

The pollen count is given as the number of grains per cubic metre and can only be a general average. The concentration can vary widely according to local conditions, even within a few hundred yards. In June and July the count can rise to 200 — which is considered to be high — but a concentration of 50 grains per cubic metre is likely to affect most sufferers. In some areas on a hot and windy day the pollen count can rise to several thousand grains per cubic metre, and along some motorways and major roads it can reach 1,000 to 5,000 grains per cubic metre. The eddy-currents set up by fast-moving traffic increase the movement of pollens in the atmosphere.

Pollen counts usually reach their peak in the mornings and evenings, especially on hot breezy days. The hay fever victim is always relieved to see the rain which settles the pollens and clears the air.

Inhalation

We all inhale airborne particles of various descriptions when we breathe. In the spring or summer these may consist mainly of pollens, even if we are in a city. Our noses filter most particles during quiet breathing, preventing pollen grains from reaching our lungs.

Pollen grains are large enough to be filtered by sufficiently healthy membranes in the nose and sinuses. Large pollen particles, from grasses for example, measure from 25-30 microns in diameter whilst trees and plants, such as the birch, or ragweed, produce finer pollens of 20 microns diameter. Even these smaller particles do not normally reach the lungs unless we become very weakened. The smaller spores from moulds have a diameter of only 3-5 microns and they are more common causes of asthmatic problems.

Nasal blockage and strenuous physical work, both of which tend to make us breathe through our mouths, may allow grains to reach the lungs and this increases the risk of asthmatic wheezes.

Any particles which get through the mucous membranes may trigger off the allergic response in a sensitized person but over-irritation at the surface may also produce excessive mucus which can become catarrhal. It is important to maintain healthy mucous membranes to prevent hay fever.

Medical treatments

Various drugs, such as antihistamines, have been devised to confront the symptoms of hay fever; and other procedures, such as desensitization, have been developed. Because they invariably deal with only a small aspect of the disorder their success has been limited.

Antihistamines. These are drugs which neutralize the histamine, thereby reducing the irritation, swelling, and constriction which it causes. They are sedative in effect and often make people feel drowsy.

Steroids are drugs used for their anti-inflammatory effects in severe forms of hay fever and asthma. They suppress the immune response, which may give short term relief to hay fever sufferers, but definitely have long-term disadvantages for their overall health. There are many unpleasant side-effects of prolonged steroid use, including blood changes and interference with the normal growth of children.

Sodium cromoglycate is a drug which was developed in the late 1960's and was found to prevent bronchospasm in asthmatics. It acts primarily by stabilizing the mast cells, so inhibiting the release of histamine. It does nothing to stop the action of histamine once it has been released. It is also used for hay fever, but it is important to take it regularly to prevent symptoms occurring. It has an excellent safety record and is the principle ingredient in some well-known anti-allergic therapies for asthma and hay fever, such as Intel. Its inclusion in eye drops has been found to relieve the irritation associated with allergic sensitivity.

Desensitization. In cases where a sensitivity to particular pollens can be determined, small purified doses of the antigen are prepared and injected on a regular basis. These stimulate the release of other antibodies which combine with the pollen protein molecules whenever they meet them in the future and prevent them reaching the IgE in the tissues. Some people find desensitizing injections helpful for a season or two, and certain reports have given a success rate as high as 70 per cent. The benefits don't last, however, and in a year or two other pollens may find their way through the body defences if nothing is done to improve the general level of health and immunity.

Vaccinations against various disabling diseases are a favourite target of medical researchers. Vaccines are believed to induce artificial immunity in much the same way as desensitizing injections. The long-term benefits of vaccination are questionable. People who have a genetic susceptibility to certain pollens may not even respond to vaccines. Furthermore, because the injected preparations of antigens bypass important defence mechanisms, such as the lymphatic barriers of pharynx and throat, they may be a cause of malfunction of the general immune system. Routine childhood vaccinations, for example, commit 30-70 per cent of the total immune capacity of the body compared with the 3-7 per cent used up in acquiring natural immunity, thus lowering already limited reserves for other crises.

Most of the commonly used drugs can give effective short-term relief and may even be life-saving where symptoms become particularly severe, especially if someone has difficulty breathing because of asthmatic spasms of the lungs, but these situations are rare and for most hay fever sufferers there are safer natural forms of treatment.

The drugs and treatment described here are only available on prescription by a medical doctor, so, if you or your child suffer from severe symptoms of hay fever, or breathing difficulty, you should consult your G.P.

A brighter future

Whilst symptomatic relief may be a very desirable short-term objective for every hay fever sufferer, it is of little value if the problem keeps recurring. Hay fever is said to have little effect on the general health, but there is no question that your general health has a lot to do with your susceptibility to hay fever.

So far I have described only *how* hay fever happens, but not *why*. To discover this we need to look at the health of the body as a whole and not merely at the intricate mechanisms of the nasal membranes. There are various factors which can undermine your health and immunity, many of them controllable, and by giving attention to them it is possible to develop a positive plan of action to reduce the misery of hay fever and enable you to begin to look forward to spring and summer with greater pleasure.

2 The Real Causes of Hay Fever

The breaking of body defences

Fascinating though they may be, the intricate biochemical mechanisms and physical changes which bring about the horror of hay fever symptoms are only part of the story. If you are to develop a progressive plan of help for yourself as a hay fever sufferer you must look beyond the immediate superficial symptoms to your general health. Symptoms may be confined to one area of the body but modern medicine is beginning to accept the view — long held by practitioners of natural therapy (alternative medicine) — that the functions of any part of the body must be seen in relation to the whole. Even though the hay fever sufferer may have a sore face and head, he or she also has feelings, and skin and blood, and digestive organs, which are all interdependent and affect the head.

Understanding the detailed mechanisms of a disease may enable chemists to develop specific drugs to modify the changes and neutralize a substance which causes an unpleasant sensation, such as histamine, but this does nothing to correct the real causes of the disorder. They are the gradual breakdown of the healthy function of the body and the progressive weakening of resistance.

Contradiction in defence

It may seem as though there is a contradiction here. Hay fever symptoms are the result of an exaggerated defensive response against the invasion of pollens, and other foreign proteins, and this would suggest that the body's protective mechanisms are more than adequate. But the fact that the invading particles have got through to the tissues means that there is a weakness in the first line of defence, the mucous membranes of the nose, throat, sinuses, and lungs. The quality and tone of the surface cells is in some way insufficient to resist the penetration of the pollens, and they fail to move them on to where they can do no harm, either in the gut or out of the body again.

The over-sensitive response of the immune system also suggests an imbalance of function there. Such inappropriate responses are the result of a breakdown of the normal immunity which can be brought about by a wide range of factors. The objective of our positive plan against hay fever is to build up your natural immunity and general well-being so that your feverish sore head and streaming nose can gradually return to normal.

Total life burden

Our health potential is determined by the burdens we accumulate as our life progresses. We start out with the genetic endowment we inherit from our parents and pick up both positive and negative attributes; some factors may strengthen us and others will be added bricks to the load we have to carry on our journey through life. Poor nutrition, suppressed illness, fatigue, stress, and other bricks of varying weight may be added to our burden. As it becomes greater, and we become less effective in bearing it, the small extra load that pollens provide may be like the camel's last straw. This book describes how to take bricks *off* your load.

Threats to health

A healthy body is well equipped to cope with most natural things to which it is exposed, pollens included. The trouble with modern life is that it poses threats to our health and well-being which can lead to sensitivity to all sorts of natural substances that normally wouldn't cause any trouble. As our resistance becomes weaker we may start to become sensitive to more and more things.

Medical science has, so far, made the mistake of suggesting that the factors which may trigger off symptoms are their cause. So, a few years ago, it was fashionable to blame 'a bug' if we felt unwell; now we suspect that we are 'allergic to something' without stopping to think why we might have become susceptible.

There is no doubt that hay fever is more common than ever before and this must, in some part, be attributed to the vicissitudes of modern life which more readily undermine our health and resistance. These include the burdensome 'bricks' of stress, inadequate rest, poor nutrition, junk foods, stimulants, many medical drugs, and air pollution; all of which have been shown to depress the functions of our immune systems. But the encouraging thing is that, although we may all be exposed to one or more of these factors at some time or other, they are at least things over which we have control. In fact, when you look at all the reasons why we may become unwell there is only a small proportion — the hereditary factors — about which we can do little and, even then, by attention to lifestyle and the adoption of health-promoting measures we can overcome most inherited weaknesses.

Hereditary factors

It has been estimated that as much as 30 per cent of our health potential is governed by genetic factors — the strengths and weaknesses we inherit from our parents, grandparents, and beyond. Just as we may inherit the features of our faces or feet, so may we be endowed a certain weakness of function in some tissue and organs. About 10 per cent of the population have a higher concentration of IgE in their tissues which means that they are more likely to suffer from hay fever and related complaints such as rhinitis or asthma. In some cases there is an inherited predisposition to produce specific antibodies, but often there is a more general sensitivity. In other words, a parent or grandparent might have had only eczema (a skin condition which is often caused by allergic sensitivities) but you could develop hay fever and asthma, with or without the skin problems.

Other disorders which can have a relationship to allergy are migraine and diabetes. If people in your family suffer from these you might be inclined to develop other sensitivities, including hay fever. Children of a parent who is diabetic, for example, are more inclined to develop low blood sugar (see page 30) because of the inherited tendency to sensitivity of the pancreas, the gland which regulates the sugar levels in our bodies.

It must be emphasized that we only inherit a *tendency* to these disorders; they are not inevitable in the way that some genetic disorders, such as haemophilia, are. Haemophilia is a condition in which wounds do not heal due to a failure of the blood clotting mechanism which is passed on by a defective chromosome in the genes of one parent. It is a defect which is there whether the victim likes it or not; but with susceptibilities, such as hay fever, the disorders only develop when you create the right environment for them to establish themselves. So, although we cannot do much about the features passed on to us, we can do a great deal to improve the efficiency of our general health and body defences by working on that 70 per cent over which we do have control. Even though you may have a family history of allergy you need not become a permanent victim of hay fever.

Whether or not there is a family tendency to allergy, such people are described as *atopic* (from the Greek *atopos*, meaning 'out of place') but hay fever and other sensitivities can develop without any genetic predisposition if we overtax or weaken our body's natural adaptive mechanisms.

Basic essentials of health

While twentieth-century science and medicine were devoting considerable skills and enormous resources to the study of disease, discovering ever more intricate details in an attempt to modify the mechanism by some chemical means, others were working quietly to determine what maintained wellness. Their territory was not the laboratory — with its test tubes, chemicals, and captive rats, mice, and monkeys — it was real people, in their normal environment, tribes in far off places who knew no disease of civilization, patients nearer home who responded to their health restoring treatments. People like the naturopaths, Henry Lindlahr and Bernarr Macfadden in America; Stanley Lief and James C. Thompson in the U.K., Maurice Blackmore in Australia; doctors in Europe, such as Max Bircher-Benner in Switzerland, and A. L. Reckeweg in Germany; and Weston A. Price, who studied the health of many primitive tribes in Central and Southern America. They were the real pioneers of health.

Basing their discoveries entirely on the observation of people in health and disease, either those they studied or those they treated (often after conventional medicine had failed) they all came, quite independently, to the same conclusion — that disease is not due to germs, or viruses, or moulds, or pollens, but to the breakdown in the natural functions of the body itself. This, they stated, was the result of poor nutrition,

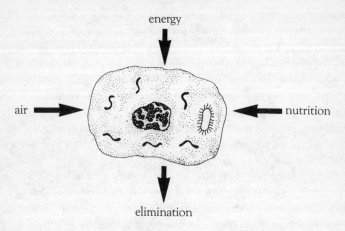

Figure 4. The basic essentials.

and poor elimination of waste products.

The body is composed of millions of cells which are all interdependent but which have basic requirements for healthy function. They need air, nutrition, energy, and adequate elimination. Without the first three they decline in vitality and without being able to eliminate waste products they will become clogged and sluggish. These are the Basic Essentials for the cells individually and collectively in the whole body.

Toxaemia theories

It was the pioneer naturopaths, in both Europe and America, who put forward the theory that the cells of our bodies will slowly but imperceptibly decline in vitality when they are not well nourished or cannot eliminate waste products efficiently. The tissues gradually accumulate a sort of sludge of impurities from body waste and the undesirable poisons which enter it with our food or air. It is now widely recognized that these toxins will damage our cells by oxidation, and interfere with essential enzymes and other biochemical functions in the body. The ability of our bodies to neutralize these poisons depends on good nutrition and their effective elimination via the skin, lungs, kidneys, and bowels.

The toxaemia theories suggest that the slow 'sludging up' of our systems creates a seedbed in which disease can easily become established.

Intestinal toxaemia

Constipation is considered to be one of the major causes of chronic and degenerative diseases. Inadequate emptying of the colon means that the rate at which impurities are absorbed from the blood is slowed down and the overflow of irritants must, therefore, be carried to the skin and other surfaces, such as the mucous membranes. The skin in turn can become sluggish and the mucous membranes may become hypersensitive to pollens and other external irritants and produce excessive catarrh.

Toxic focus

The burden of poisonous chemicals in the body may also be increased by inadequately resolved or suppressed infections in areas such as the teeth or tonsils. A small area of unresolved infection in the body is known as a toxic focus. A chronic abcess in the gums, or infected tonsillar tissue may seep poison into the system which can interfere with normal body chemistry and keep it in a constant state of poor health.

A toxic focus can often be treated by diet and properly directed herbal or homoeopathic medicine, but may occasionally need removal by surgery if these methods fail. When this is done, attention must be given to the general health and nutrition to help the body to restore its normal internal balance.

Chemical poisons

Our bodies are subjected to a wide range of chemical intrusions from food additives and environmental pollution. Some chemicals used in the home may cause problems for sensitive individuals. Aluminium, for example, is a toxic metal which may enter the blood from food cooked in aluminium utensils. Aluminium interferes with some enzyme functions in the body and may often aggravate allergies.

Dental fillings, consisting of an amalgam of mercury and silver which has been in use for many years, may cause mercury levels to rise in the body. Mercury has been shown by researchers in the U.S.A. to suppress the white blood cells in the immune response. Mercury also reduces tissue vitamin C levels.

The amount of toxic metals in the body can be measured, and such toxic elements can be neutralized and removed by nutritional methods. In severe cases of allergy where the dental fillings are found to be contributing to the disorder, careful dental replacement of the amalgam may be necessary.

Low blood sugar

Hay fever often comes as an added torment to people who are already somewhat fatigued or bothered by other allergic disorders. This is because their energy levels always seem to be falling. Over several million years the human body has evolved an efficient energy producing metabolism. In the last one hundred years or so the changes in eating habits which mankind has imposed upon itself have made impossible demands on the adaptive powers of the human digestive system.

Without doubt the biggest change has been in our consumption of sugar. From being obtained by gradual digestion and absorption from fruits, berries, nuts, and grains (all protein food is ultimately converted to sugar for energy) it has been changed to a highly refined concentrated pseudo-food which is absorbed too rapidly, with the consequent disruption of the energy physiology.

The result is a condition known as functional hypoglycaemia which is now so prevalent that it has been described by naturopath Martin L. Budd, in his book *Low Blood Sugar* (Thorsons, 1981), as the 'twentieth century epidemic'. Functional hypoglycaemia is the basis of many allergies and conditions as diverse as depression, arthritis and migraine.

The sugar energy paradox

When sugar in any form is consumed the sugar level in the blood rises but is not available for energy until the pancreas, a gland lying below the stomach, secretes insulin. The insulin breaks the sugar down into a form which the body can use for energy, but if there is repeated absorption of refined sugar the pancreas becomes sensitive and produces too much insulin which quickly uses up the available energy reserves. If this pattern continues over many months or years a chronic state of low blood sugar, or functional hypoglycaemia, becomes established and can give rise to the wide range of disorders which occur when the body's energy and immunity are impaired. The problem may be made worse by other stimulants, such as caffeine in coffee and nicotine in cigarettes, and is associated with deficiencies of such minerals and trace elements as magnesium and zinc.

Sugar manufacturers promote the energy-giving properties of their products, but the paradox is that, although chemically it provides energy, physiologically that energy does not last.

Dr Carl C. Pfeiffer, Director of the Brain Bio Center in New York, has found that hypoglycaemics generally have higher tissue histamine levels than normal controls. This makes them more vulnerable to histamine releasing processes following pollen exposure. I have found that many of my patients with allergies and food sensitivities are hypoglycaemic. The introduction of a sugar-free diet with adequate protein — especially from slowly absorbed foods, such as grains and pulses — with appropriate supplements will correct the disorder.

Food allergy

Some people are sensitive to a wide variety of foods or certain chemicals in them. They are said to have food allergy, although, in many cases, this may not be true allergy but an intolerance for a variety of reasons ranging from an inability to digest certain constituents of a food item — for example, the lactose in cows' milk — to a physiological response to chemicals — such as caffeine in coffee.

Intolerance may develop to a wide variety of constituents in foods, particularly chemicals used for preserving or colouring them, and the residues of fertilizers and sprays applied during growing. Naturally occurring compounds in foods have also been found to cause problems for very sensitive individuals. One of the principal trouble makers is the yellow colouring agent Tartrazine. With other related compounds it may precipitate rashes, rhinitis, and behavioural problems in children.

Chemicals in food

Supporters of chemicals on or in our food take delight in countering criticism of their fare with tales of the poisons to be found naturally in many foods. Their argument does not diminish the danger to sensitive individuals of food additives, nor their cumulative threat to the health of us all.

Among the preservatives the most widely used are a group known as the sulphites. One of these, sulphur dioxide, is used to preserve fruits and vegetables, and another, sodium metabisulphite, is also found in fruit juices, soft drinks, sausages, potato crisps and many other everyday foods. The sulphites were found to induce spasms of the bronchi — the smaller tubes which branch off the main airways into the lungs — in children who were asthmatic. As little as 10-15mg can elicit an adverse reaction, and the risk for some individuals can be appreciated when you realize that one handful of dried apricots can contain 200mg.

Allergic manifestations have also been noted after taking salicylates. These chemicals are the basis of drugs such as aspirin, but they also occur naturally in many plant foods. If you have a sensitivity to aspirin you may also be upset, in a less obvious way, by such foods as apples, apricots, avocados, cherries, grapefruit, pineapple, rhubarb, broad beans, beetroot, broccoli, cucumber, spinach, sweet corn, mushrooms, onions, tea, most alcohol, almonds, Brazil nuts, peanuts, sesame seeds, honey, liquorice, and yeast containing foods. That is a depressingly long list containing many otherwise nutritious foods, so do not expect to have to exclude them all. Most hay fever sufferers can tolerate the salicylates in these foods because they are buffered by the other natural ingredients.

Other food theories

Certain other nutritional causes of hay fever have been put forward, such as incompatible food combinations and disturbances of fatty acid metabolism.

Food combining

Dr W.H. Hay, the creator of the Hay Diet, suggested that, because they require different digestive juices, foods such as starches and proteins should not be eaten in the same meal. When they are they may create biochemical imbalances which lay the foundation for many illnesses.

In *Food Combining for Health* by Doris Grant and Jean Joice (Thorsons, 1984) Dr Hay is quoted as saying that by suitable selection of foods 'the hay fever sufferer can so change his body chemistry that he can bury his face in his former *betes noir*, no matter what this happens to be, without a single sneeze.' The Hay Diet, in which incompatible food classes are eaten at different meals, is, therefore, another way of reducing the body's biochemical imbalance and minimizing the toxic burden. It will be considered in more detail in Chapter 4.

Prostaglandins

A group of regulatory hormones which have attracted increasing attention by biochemists in recent years are the prostaglandins. They were so named because they were first isolated from seminal fluid and were believed to be produced in the prostate gland, which manufactures this fluid in the male. Prostaglandins are, in fact, produced and utilized by most cells in the body.

There are several types of prostaglandin, labelled PGE_1, PGE_2, and PGE_3. Some of these are pro-inflammatory and others, such as PGE_1, inhibit inflammation. PGE_1 is low in allergic individuals, and hay fever may be just one of a number of disorders in which the metabolism of essential fatty acids, from which prostaglandins are derived, may be disturbed. Essential fatty acids (EFA's) are a group of fats which must be included in our diet for healthy function of the immune system. They are an integral part of the basic health diet described in Chapter 4.

There have always been fashions in diets and 'wonder foods' for a wide variety of ailments, and hay fever is no exception. What works for one person may not be so helpful for another but, if it is harmless, it is worth a try. There is a grain of good sense in many of these ideas and their potential for help will be that much better if you can get the basics right.

I have introduced just some of the many factors, both nutritional and environmental, which can disturb body chemistry, impair the complex energy producing and defensive processes, and interfere with elimination. There are other important bricks which add to the burden, too, such as poor posture and emotional stress. We shall consider all the factors which may have any bearing on your hay fever but, if you are suffering now, you will need an immediate plan of action.

3 A Plan of Action

Taking control

The marvellous thing about biological systems, such as our bodies, is that their functions can be accelerated and improved. This is because we have a reserve, both mentally and physically, which is seldom fully developed. Since many people's metabolisms are working at well below their optimum potential, this may merely mean encouraging it to do what it should be doing anyway. But, whatever your starting point, there is certainly scope for improvement by applying various strategies which are described in this book. Positive action on different fronts, such as nutrition, exercise, adequate rest, physical stimuli, and visualization can definitely increase health and resistance.

You may shut yourself indoors with windows closed throughout the height of the summer, and avoid exposing yourself too greatly to the pollens, but by breathing exercises, tonic bathing, and mental imagery, you can actually improve the efficiency with which the nose, sinuses, and lungs resist the external irritants.

Potentiating health

Even passive measures, such as excluding from the diet the foods and drinks which reduce resistance, will help out. By adopting a diet rich in nutrients and using appropriate natural supplements, you can actually enhance the function of the immune system.

You can swallow antihistamine drugs, or inhale decongestant sprays, and go around in a fog of lethargy with thickened, chronically swollen nasal membranes, or you can undertake a short cleansing fast, and use some of the herbal or homoeopathic remedies which are available to promote healthy function. You have the power to potentiate your health.

Making the choice

You also have a choice. You can seek short-term relief — and you may find it, only to have to go on looking again and again while you slowly decline in health — or you can take positive action now and start on a programme which will rectify the real causes of your hay fever. Of course it will take time to overcome the problem completely, probably several seasons, but you can expect definite signs of improvement quite quickly if you adopt a comprehensive approach, attending to the various health needs of your body.

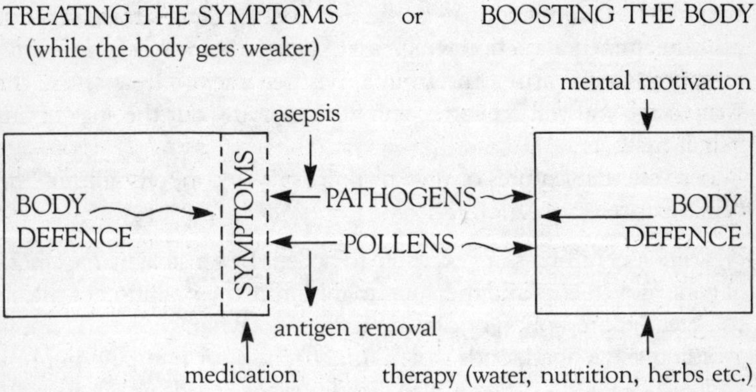

TREATING THE SYMPTOMS   or   BOOSTING THE BODY
  (while the body gets weaker)

Figure 5. Hay fever — the choice.

It will also require effort on your part. Many people take their health for granted expecting the body to go on working and defending itself without any real care and attention. It may seem a hackneyed analogy, but if your car starts faltering or shows signs of rust you take steps to rectify it; you get the engine serviced and give it an oil change or rub down the rust and put on protective paint. But when hay fever symptoms start people still expect to keep going on as before and try to mask the symptoms. It's like putting in ear plugs when driving, so that you don't hear the clattering of the engine, or covering up the rust patches without using any primer. People may take the view that it shouldn't be necessary to think about their health; it should be maintained automatically and it is the responsibility of medical science to provide an easy answer to any problems. I hope that you are not one of these people.

You have in your hands proposals for personal action which may not be all plain sailing but they will be effective. Unlike a car the human body does have powers of self-repair provided it gets the right raw materials for the job, and it is those powers that our hay fever treatment plans to promote.

Immediate action

The comprehensive approach to hay fever really needs to be introduced several months before the summer pollens start arriving, but even if you are in the throes of an acute attack you can institute immediate action which may give you some relief. No matter how firmly established the trouble has become, or how severe the symptoms, you will get some help from carrying out the suggestions I shall make here.

The essential features of your plan are prevention, promotion, and perseverance:

Prevention of unnecessary exposure to pollens by sensible management of your movements and measures to minimize the pollution of the air you breathe. Prevention by care in the choice of what you eat and drink, avoiding the refined foods which undermine your natural immunity and reduce your resistance, also avoiding those foods which increase the toxic load of the tissues, producing excessive catarrh. Prevention of undue exhaustion and destructive emotions through adequate rest, a positive outlook and the avoidance of stress.

Promotion of vitality by using wholesome foods to provide the body with the optimum nutrition it requires for building good resistance. Promotion of strong healthy mucous membranes by providing good quality nutritional supplements, using vitamins, minerals, and trace elements, which have been shown to play a vital role in cell functions and natural immunity. Promotion of better circulation and drainage to nasal and sinus membranes and lungs, using simple hydrotherapy procedures available in your own home. Promotion of clearer airways by improved breathing and regular exercise. Promotion of resistance by well-tried herbal and homoeopathic medicines.

Perseverance is required in the application of all that you undertake in your efforts to regain health. Perseverance with the short fasts and cleansing diet programmes which will, given a chance, provide more effective relief from the nasal congestion and irritation than any other single measure. Perseverance with a sensible basic diet to prevent the build up of catarrh and to sustain good energy levels. Perseverance with herbs and supplements which, unlike drugs, do not give immediate symptomatic relief, but slowly improve the vitality of the body and the integrity of specific areas, like the nasal membranes, to prevent the hypersensitive reactions.

Keeping the pollens at bay

If you are already suffering some symptoms of hay fever you may consider it's a bit late to avoid exposure, but remember each time you inhale more pollens which penetrate the membranes, a fresh sequence of histamine secretion will be initiated. The reaction may not be as pronounced as to the initial exposure but it will be enough to perpetuate the symptoms.

Generally the dry breezy days are the most difficult. Morning and early evening tend to be the worst. Flowering plants and grasses release more pollens at these times and their concentration in the atmosphere is likely to be greater. Stay indoors if you can, in the mornings and evenings particularly, and if possible keep the windows closed.

Even if you live in a town there is likely to be a high concentration of pollen in the air, not only blown in from the surrounding countryside but locally generated from trees, gardens, and parks. Try to time your shopping trips and other outings to avoid peak pollen times or, better still, do them on rainy days.

Keep lawns around you well trimmed and flowerbeds and pathways well weeded. Wild grasses grow quickly to seed in well matured beds and derelict corners. Pull them out by the roots to prevent regrowth.

An air conditioner may filter some of the larger pollen particles but any finer ones will get through. Ionizers may be helpful. They increase the number of negative ions in the atmosphere which attract pollens

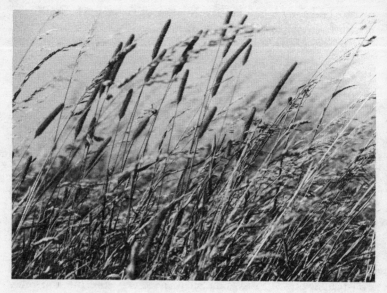

Blowing in the wind (on a breezy summer day grasses release millions of pollen grains).

and settle them so that they are less likely to be inhaled. There are some ionizers available combined with air filters, and ionizers for use in cars can be helpful. For more details about ionizers and their benefits turn to page 137.

Rainy weather brings blessed relief to hay fever victims but may well be followed by renewed vigour in the growth of plants. The pollen count tends to be much lower on the coast, especially when the wind is blowing off the sea, so a summer visit to the seaside may be a good way of keeping the pollens at bay.

Motoring

Be particularly careful when you are driving because grassy banks on country roads and motorways are a rich source of pollen. Do not use the air intake for ventilation; use instead the recycle device if you have one.

It pays to prevent sneezes. One sneeze while travelling at 60 miles an hour can cause you to be unsighted for over 40 yards. If you feel a sneeze coming on, firm pressure with the side of the finger immediately under the nose may help to abort it.

Clearing the congestion

One of the simplest and oldest forms of treatment is hydrotherapy — the use of water in various ways to promote the health and function of the body. These are more fully dealt with in Chapter 9 which explains various tonic measures, but there are a number of simple ways in which water therapy can help the hay fever sufferer.

Packs and compresses can be used in the treatment of feverish conditions and to promote eliminative functions. Enemas are a useful adjunct to a general cleansing programme, and inhalations have proved their worth for the relief of stuffy nose and sinuses. But you can get considerable relief by the simple expedient of cold splashing or sponging of the face and throat area.

Cold water is tonic in its action on the skin. It encourages contraction of the small blood vessels in the vicinity sending stagnant blood away from the area, reducing local congestion, and encouraging better drainage of the histamine from the tissues.

Splash your face and eyes repeatedly with cold water for two or three minutes every hour or two if you are suffering, but try to do it several times a day as a general tonic measure, even if your hay fever is not too bad. Remember, the less congested and catarrhal you are, the less the likelihood of severe discomfort if you do inhale some pollens.

Sore throats may be relieved by cold compresses and more detailed directions for their application are given in Chapter 9.

Water sniffing is found to be very soothing for people with raw, burning nasal membranes. Cold water is sniffed up into the nostrils and allowed to run back into the pharynx or blown out again. This may be repeated several times. The cooling effect is soothing and it may relieve some of the congestion and remove pollen particles. Water sniffing should not be performed more than once or twice a day, as excessive irrigation of nasal membranes washes away natural protective secretions.

Steam inhalations can be used to relieve stuffy catarrhal tubes. Position your face over a bowl of boiling water and cover it with a towel and inhale deeply. A few drops of a herbal mixture of aromatic oils, such as pine, wintergreen, and eucalyptus, increase the benefit. Most chemists and health food stores sell useful combinations of these oils.

The role of diet

There are various short and longer term dietary programmes which can greatly relieve the acute symptoms of hay fever. The food we eat has a considerable influence on the function and resistance of our bodies. Some foods and drinks may encourage the production of excessive amounts of catarrh; some may deplete our reserves of essential defensive vitamins and minerals, such as vitamin C, or calcium; others may upset our energy metabolism and lead to chronic fatigue with increased susceptibility to infections and allergies.

It isn't usually sufficient, however, just to avoid one or two food items and expect to get better without attention to other factors. Patients often report to me that they have cut out this or that food, because they had heard that it was harmful, but felt no better for doing so. Any avoidance of normal food items can only really help in the context of a total health programme.

Some foods to avoid

There are some foods and drinks which may increase the probability of hay fever symptoms, and you will benefit by their immediate reduction or exclusion from your diet. The trouble makers are quite often commonplace items which many people consume every day. The reasons they cause problems can vary from actual allergy (relatively rare with foods) to intolerance because of the lack of the necessary enzymes to digest them. Some foods and drinks stimulate the secretion of excessive amounts of insulin, which lowers the blood sugar level, and there are others which contain chemicals, such as salicylates, which raise the blood levels of these substances closer to the threshold so that reactions to allergens become more likely in sensitive people.

In Chapter 4 we shall look more closely at the difficulties these foods may cause but, meanwhile, you should start to exclude or reduce the following items from your diet:

Exclude   Cow's milk and milk products, such as cheese, cream, butter. Sugar, sweets, chocolates, and artificial sweeteners. Coffee, tea, soft drinks, especially cola beverages.

Reduce   Starchy foods, especially those made with
                            white flour or white rice. Alcoholic beverages,
                            especially those with high sugar content, such
                            as wines, beers, and sherry.

If that sounds rather restrictive don't worry; there are plenty of appetizing
alternatives and the Basic Health Diet on page 55 is full of positive
suggestions.

Eating for health

Whilst you must avoid the foods and drinks which cause problems
it is equally important to provide the body with the right raw materials
to develop and maintain peak energy and adequate resistance to
allergens. This will be considered in more detail in the diet chapters
but a few guidelines at this stage will help you to begin your health
programme more effectively.

One of the best ways to reduce tissue acidity and catarrh is to increase
the proportion of alkaline-forming foods. These are mainly fruits and
vegetables, and they have the greatest biological value when eaten raw.
Start by making at least one meal a day predominently raw food, perhaps
a mixed salad served with baked jacket potato or crisp bread, and some
fresh fruit to follow.

Soon you can introduce fresh fruits with your breakfast and increase
the proportion over a week or two until the breakfast is mainly fruit
and nuts or seeds. This reduces the intake of the starchy foods of which
breakfasts are so commonly composed, and allows the body to continue
what is considered to be a normal cleansing phase in the early hours
of the day.

Your evening meal may be a savoury dish with a selection of vegetables
followed by a fruit or other non-milky dessert.

Cleansing and fasting

When you are accustomed to basic changes in your
diet you may feel ready to undertake a short fast or cleansing programme.
In fact, when hay fever symptoms become acute, there is less inclination
to eat so it is a good opportunity to stick to a diet of fresh fruit or fruit
juices. A fast or raw food diet is also one of the most effective ways
of relieving acute hay fever. The special Fast Relief Plan for hay fever,
described on page 171 incorporates the principles of fasting with light

diet and supplements to give rapid alleviation of acute symptoms.

When our bodies undergo a crisis, whether locally or generally, there is increased activity and heat as it channels all its resources to the area under threat. Fever and inflammation are indications of body defence at work, burning up toxic waste. Eating excessively simply slows down that process and the energy needed for cleansing is largely diverted to the digestion. Witholding food allows the body to resolve its problems and the cooling raw foods help to take the heat out of the situation.

Detailed instructions for fasts and cleansing diets are given in Chapter 5.

Plant power

Plants, which can wreak such havoc with the respiratory systems of hay fever victims through the action of their pollens, also have the power to heal. Extracts of various medicinal herbs can be used to boost the resistance, soothe inflamed surfaces and relieve congested sinuses or wheezy bronchial tubes.

Infinitesimal quantities of some medicinal plants and mineral substances may exert dramatic changes for the better using the homoeopathic system of treatment. Homoeopathic medicines are prepared by diluting and succussing medicinal substances many times to such a degree that they cannot be detected. The power of the medicine is believed to be exerted by some subtle frequency. The most beneficial effect is obtained when the remedy is carefully matched to the patient's individual symptoms, not just the physical ones, such as runny nose or itchy eyes, but the whole personality complex of the person. There are, however, some standard homoeopathic medicines of lower dilution which can relieve the severe symptoms.

The number after the name of the remedy refers to the potency of the medicine and you may obtain it as small tablets which should be dissolved in the mouth every three to four hours. They must be used at times when there has been no other food, drink, or toothpaste in the mouth for at least one hour. These many cancel the power of the remedy.

Arsenicum album 6 is suitable for a person who experiences a pricking and burning sensation in throat and eyes, with streaming catarrh.

Pulsatilla 6 would be indicated for congested sinus and stuffy nose, with catarrh that doesn't clear easily. After taking it for a while you may be able to blow out more old mucus.

Biochemic tissue salts are minerals made up in homoeopathic dilution which can assist the clearing of congestion or inflammation in the nasal membranes. A useful combination for hay fever and rhinitis is available from health food stores.

Short-term strategies

These measures are just some of the well-tried strategies available to you which may bring effective relief to your suffering sinuses without side-effects. There are many other measures you can introduce over the coming weeks and months.

Dealing with hay fever calls for concerted action, not just through the pollen season, but throughout the year. Remember that the general health of your body has the major influence on the way you cope when the crisis comes. Hay fever doesn't happen regardless. To get a grip it needs a body which is over sensitized, catarrhally clogged, fatigued, and depressed both mentally and immunologically.

Ideally, you should introduce protective measures early in the year, cleansing the system, clearing catarrhal encumbrance, providing good elimination, and building up resistance with herbs, such as Echinacea, and supplements, such as vitamin C. These will be described fully in later chapters.

It is no longer necessary to turn to drugs for the relief of hay fever. Thousands of people have been able to alleviate and eradicate their hay fever using the methods described in this book, methods which are often based on age-old principles but are right up to date clinically and scientifically in their application.

4 *Food — for Better and for Worse*

Healthy eating to beat hay fever

Sufferers from hay fever will no doubt feel that there is an inevitability about the arrival of their symptoms with the spring and summer. We often describe them as 'victims of hay fever' — I have used the term myself in this book — which implies a helplessness against the condition. But this is far from being the case. There is a wide range of self-help measures which can be adopted.

Of all the positive steps you can take to overcome hay fever, probably the most effective — and certainly the one over which you have most control — is the modification of your eating and drinking habits. Food has both positive and negative effects on our health. On the plus side it provides nourishment and energy for our body functions, being especially important to the maintenance of adequate immunity. On the other hand, if of poor quality, over-refined, or loaded with additives, pesticides, and fertilizer residues, it can be responsible for declining vitality and an increasing burden of poisons to the system. In other words, food can make your hay fever better, but it can also make it very much worse.

Making food work for you

You can use your diet to influence your health in several important ways:

- to provide nourishment of sufficiently high quality and adequate quantity

- to increase the intake of vital nutrients
- to avoid excessively processed food and especially the 'junk' foods
- to rest the digestion, when appropriate, to encourage the healing process (e.g., with controlled diets or fasting).

Using these ground rules you are in a position to review your eating habits to make very real progress towards eradicating your hay fever.

The essential features of healthy food are that it should be:

- as fresh as possible and as near as possible to its natural state
- unrefined and free from chemical additives and residues of pesticides and fertilizers.

Apart from providing quality food for your body energy and repair, you may use the modern knowledge of nutrition to potentiate the process of recovery. Certain nutrients play a vital role in body defence mechanisms, and it is essential to ensure that they are adequately provided by the food you eat.

Finally, as I have already intimated, some everyday foods can contribute to the misery of hay fever for reasons which we shall consider more fully later in this chapter.

Before describing the Basic Diet it is worth looking at the principles upon which it has been developed. These are universally regarded as the fundamentals of healthy nutrition.

Wholefood

The relevance of food to your health was recognized over 2,000 years ago by Hippocrates, the Father of Medicine, whose frequently quoted statement 'Let your food be your medicine and your medicine be your food' is still appropriate in modern times, but needs embellishment with the proviso 'Don't let food be your poison!'

Hay fever was virtually unknown until about 150 years ago, and it may be significant that it is since that time that the consumption of sugar has risen and the practice of putting chemicals on the land to boost crop production, spraying plants with chemicals to control pests, and adding chemicals in the processing of food to preserve or colour it has increased to staggering proportions. More than sixty years ago some pioneer naturopaths and a few doctors pointed out the dangers of artificial additives and chemical sprays and the importance of natural food to the maintenance of health. Now the potential health hazards of modern agricultural practices are more widely known, and the medical and scientific evidence of intolerance to many food additives and chemical residues is accumulating daily. The inferior nutritional quality of foods which have been refined and heavily processed has also been demonstrated in numerous experiments.

In the 1940s the term *wholefood* was coined to define food which is grown without the use of chemical fertilizers or pesticides, and processed only sufficiently to be made palatable, without removal of the most nutritious parts, such as the germ of the wheat or rice. It must also be free of chemical dyes, preservatives, and emulsifiers (which are added to make fatty foods stay soft and easy to spread). (Vegetable based ingredients, such as soya lecithin, are used without harm to the consumer.)

Health begins in the soil

The health of humans, animals, and plants, all depends on a healthy soil and pollution-free environment. If quality is impaired at any point in the food chain, from the soil to our stomachs, we will eventually suffer.

It may not be sufficient for you to select natural foods if they have been grown in deficient soil. Intensive farming methods are creating deficiencies of some essential minerals and trace elements. In a United States study, carried out in the Mid-Western states, 1,000 crop samples were analysed for basic minerals, such as copper, sodium, calcium, and manganese. Over a period of four years the mineral levels declined by as much as 68 per cent for copper, with major drops in the levels of sodium (55 per cent), calcium (41 per cent), manganese (34 per cent), and iron (26 per cent).

Food which has been organically grown, using natural manures and proper crop rotation to replenish the soil structure, is likely to have a better biological quality, so try to obtain it when you can. It may not be easy to get hold of and it may cost a little more but it is worth the effort to reduce the total burden of poisonous chemicals your body has to deal with. People with allergies need to make every effort to reduce their sensitivities.

Sunlight value

One of the great twentieth century pioneers of healthy nutrition, Dr Max Bircher-Benner, wrote in his book *The Prevention of Incurable Disease* (James Clark & Co. Ltd., 1959) of the importance of abundant fresh raw foods in the diet. The energy potentials of raw foods are greater since they contain much of the vitality of the living plant. Dr Bircher-Benner, who founded the famous Bircher-Benner Clinic in Zurich, and was also the originator of muesli, called this the 'sunlight value' of the food.

Opinions vary as to the proportion of raw food we should have in our basic diet. It may range from 60-80 per cent of the total food intake, and depends partly on our build. Tall, thin people tend to have difficulty extracting energy from high cellulose, fibrous food, and need rather more cooked foods, grains, and proteins. The shorter, stockily built individuals have more intestinal surface area and can thrive on plenty of salads, raw vegetables and fruit.

Another way of ensuring adequate raw food of maximum nutritional value is by sprouting grains. This is usually done in special equipment which can be used in your own kitchen (see page 58). Your intake of raw foods may also be increased by serving *crudités* — small portions of raw vegetables, such as carrot, cauliflower, and spring onions — with a tasty tofu dip (see page 177) as starters to each main meal. More fresh fruit desserts is another way of meeting this requirement.

Fibre

The indigestible cellulose portion of fruits, vegetables, grains, and seeds, is a vital ingredient of a healthy diet. Because it does not provide any immediate nutriment, physicians and nutritionists disregarded it for many years. The price was an increasing incidence of the very disorders they thought it aggravated, such as intestinal cancer, diverticulosis, and irritable bowel syndrome. The value of fibre as a preventative of intestinal toxaemia was recognized over 100 years ago, but it was not until the 1950s when Surgeon Captain T.L. Cleave, and D.P. Burkitt, published their studies of the health of some African tribes, that its value was more widely recognized medically. They noticed that the stools of native tribesmen, living on a diet of grains and local vegetables, were bulkier than those of Europeans who were living on refined carbohydrates with an especially high intake of sugar. The incidence of many degenerative diseases, such as coronary thrombosis, diabetes, and the intestinal disorders, was also much less in the tribesmen.

Fibre helps to prevent constipation, thereby increasing the absorption of the impurities from the intestinal walls. It also provides a matrix for the lactic acid bacteria which maintain healthy colons and provide some of our vitamin requirements. Fibre in food also absorbs excess fluids and carries away surplus fat, so maintaining a healthier balance in the body.

When you introduce more vegetables, fruit, and grains, there should be sufficient fibre in your diet and it should not be necessary to take extra bran, for example, which can interfere with the absorption of iron and calcium. Don't be fooled by commercially processed foods which pander to the current fashion by adding a bit of bran or leaving out some sugar, whilst still containing other undesirable ingredients. If in doubt seek the advice of your health food store owner who has to apply high standards to the choice of the foods he sells.

Everyday foods which make trouble

Some staple and regularly consumed foods and drinks can make your hay fever worse. This may be because they aggravate an existing allergy or cannot be digested properly (e.g., milk), or because they contain chemicals which upset your system when used in too great a quantity (e.g., coffee), or because the form in which they are consumed is unsuitable for your body (e.g., sugar).

Sugar, milk, and coffee, together with some other everyday foods, are probably mainly responsible for the enormous increase in the incidence of hay fever and other allergies. Some of these items are consumed in considerable quantities, especially by children. There are definite physiological reasons why they cause problems on such a wide scale, but they are all things which people find difficult to reduce or exclude from their diet. Fortunately there are satisfactory and enjoyable alternatives, and those who have succeeded in making a change have noticed a distinct improvement in their hay fever.

The milk debate

Milk is widely promoted as an essential and nutritious food. On analysis it does contain important nutrients — protein, fat, and minerals, especially calcium — and it is, indeed, a valuable food when taken in moderation by those who can digest it sufficiently well. Unfortunately, many people are unable to do this, principally, because, as a species, we do not have sufficient lactase enzyme to break down the lactose in cow's milk.

Lactose is the disaccharide sugar in milk. It is composed of two monosaccharides, glucose and galactose, which combine to form the disaccharide. The disaccharide must be broken down into its two monosaccharides before it can be absorbed from our intestines. The breakdown is performed by lactase, which is active in the upper part of our digestive tract from infancy, but from the age of about one to four it declines in efficiency. Lactose which has not been properly broken down in the small intestine moves on to the colon, or large intestine, where the undigested material is acted upon by bacteria. This causes gas and water to accumulate in the colon which leads to bloating and discomfort, and it increases the absorption of other irritants.

Some infants are born with a lactase deficiency and are unable to tolerate any milk products. They must be given a special formula food. Lactase can be obtained from a chemist and may improve the efficiency of milk digestion but it doesn't overcome some of the other problems with milk.

The ratio of fats to proteins and their quality, also makes milk rather indigestible and many infants who are weaned onto cow's milk at an early age may also develop antibodies to the proteins which can, when other factors lower the level of health, lead to a milk allergy. One of the principal effects of milk allergy or intolerance is excess catarrh.

When my booklet *Diets to Help Hay Fever and Asthma* was first published, nearly twenty years ago, the Milk Marketing Board, ever vigilant of any threat to their interests, asked me to substantiate my recommendation to exclude milk from the diet of hay fever sufferers. At that time I could only cite the sheer weight of clinical evidence; when my pateints cut out milk products their allergies and catarrh improved. Since then numerous studies have identified milk as a cause of catarrhal and other allergic manifestations, such as asthma and eczema.

The more catarrhal you are the more the likelihood of a streaming nose or stuffy sinuses when the pollens start flying. An essential first step is to stop using cow's milk in your diet either as a drink or on breakfast cereals, and to review carefully other ways in which you may consume it, for example, in tea, coffee, cocoa, butter, cheese, ice cream, scrambled eggs, custards, puddings, trifles, and flans. Because it is such a convenient and widely used food it may seem impossible to exclude it completely and this may only be necessary if you have a definite allergy to milk. With a true allergy even a small amount of milk will, in very sensitive individuals, trigger off an adverse reaction. Most of us, however, can tolerate small amounts of milk in cooking, or baking, or in cottage or low fat cheeses and yogurt.

To minimize the mucus which aggravates your hay fever, however, you should try to eliminate all cow's milk products for a few months prior to and during the season. Later, when your health improves you may be able to tolerate moderate amounts of milk in low-fat preparations, such as those mentioned above. Fortunately, there are several reasonable and equally nutritious alternatives to cow's milk:

Goat's or sheep's milks are usually well tolerated by allergic and catarrhal people. The proteins and minerals in goat's milk are closer to those of human breast milk. The proteins are also of better quality than those in cow's milk, and the fat is more easily digested and assimilated. Goat's and sheep's milk taste different and children may be resistant to them at first. Some children who are sensitive to cow's milk may also react to goat's milk but should be able to tolerate sheep's milk.

Soya milk is now widely available from health food stores and grocery stores in cartons. Use the sugar-free variety. Soya milk is rich in protein and is a good source of calcium and is at least as nutritious as cow's milk.

Tofu is a soya preparation, fermented by the lactic acid process (similar to yogurt), which is a valuable protein food. It is available as a tasteless curd which can be used instead of milk to make flans, sauces, dressings, and desserts. It is an excellent addition to savoury dishes and stews.

Almond milk is prepared by mixing finely ground almonds in a blender with a small amount of water. They can be mixed to a creamy consistency, for fruit salads or dressings, or more thinly, to use as a milk.

Yogurt is prepared by the action of lactic acid bacteria on milk. The bacteria, usually *Lactobacillus bulgaricus*, break down the solids in milk to a readily digestible form. The lactobacilli help to build up the intestinal flora — the colonies of healthy bacteria in the colon which provide us with some nutrients and prevent constipation. The lactic acid they produce destroys the putrefactive bacteria which cause fermentation. Yogurt is, therefore, a nutritious and valuable food for colon cleanliness. Natural yogurt also inhibits histamine production. Goat's milk yogurt is preferable. Take it plain or with a natural fruit flavouring, but without sugar.

Whey is the liquid left after curd cheese or cottage cheese is made. Don't pour it away but mix it in to the cheese if it separates out. In Scandinavia and many parts of Europe whey is used regularly. It is a valuable source of calcium, iron, vitamins B_1 and B_2, and is low in fat.

Cottage cheese and other low fat cheeses such as Ricotta (Italian sheep's milk cheese) are usually an acceptable and nutritious food and may be used in place of the harder, more fatty cheeses.

Sugar

The rate at which scientific evidence is accumulating to confirm the health hazards of too much sugar makes it a strong candidate for a Government Health Warning similar to that for cigarette smoking. Sugar is ubiquitous in the diet, not only as a direct sweetener in tea, coffee, or on cereals, but as an ingredient of many other foods. Here are some of the foods and treats which contain sugar:

> cakes, bread, biscuits;
> sweets, chocolates, desserts;
> instant beverages, wines, cordials, cola drinks;
> baked beans, and other canned foods;
> sauces, dressings, and ketchups.

Sugar is big business and millions are spent in trying to persuade us to eat more, and, after years of warnings by leading naturopaths and nutritionists, the government's National Advisory Committee on Nutritional Education (NACNE) has at last recommended a reduction in its consumption, mainly because it is a cause of tooth decay, obesity, and heart disease. Sugar also contributes to many other problems, including diabetes, diverticulitis, irritable bowel syndrome, gall stones, and, most notably for the allergic hay fever sufferer, reactive hypoglycaemia, or low blood sugar.

How can too much sugar cause low blood sugar? Most forms of sugar are absorbed too rapidly, and gradually your metabolism can become over-sensitive to it. This results in secretion of too much insulin which uses up the sugar too rapidly, causing energy deficiencies which undermine your body's defences. Experiments have shown that sugar reduces the immune white cell count. Sugar also leaches certain minerals from the blood and contributes to deficiencies.

The highly concentrated form of refined sugar, taken regularly by many people, is most unnatural. A person drinking five cups of tea or coffee a day, each with a teaspoonful of sugar, would need to consume four apples to get that amount. The average weekly consumption of sugar would require sixteen pounds of sugarbeet to produce it. To take that amount of sugar in the way for which our metabolism was designed we would need to chew our way through all that sugarbeet. Some people make their energy levels rise and fall repeatedly throughout the day by constant sugary snacks, stimulants such as caffeine, and inadequate meals. Sugar gives quick relief to hunger but provides no lasting nourishment. So children who snack on sweets and starchy foods tend to miss meals and develop deficiencies. Likewise the bibbers who imbibe a 'liquid lunch'; they are effectively inscribing their own prescription for deficiency and disease.

Curtailing the sweet tooth

A craving for something sweet is a very basic human condition which arises from the need for immediate energy. This can be offset, to some extent, by eating savoury unrefined foods which are broken down more slowly by your digestive system and absorbed only gradually so that they go on providing energy for many hours.

Try to exclude from your diet anything which contains sugar and substitute savoury foods such as nuts, seeds, and grains. Instead of biscuits with your morning or afternoon beverage, have snacks of a few handsful of sunflower seeds, which are a highly nutritious protein food and will be much more sustaining. Pumpkin seeds are also an agreeable alternative.

Fresh fruit, or even dried fruits, are acceptable additions to foods as sweeteners. They contain fructose (fruit sugar) which is absorbed more slowly and is less likely to precipitate the over-hasty insulin response which glucose and sucrose cause. Dried fruits, such as raisins and sultanas, may be used in cooking and baking instead of sugar.

Honey contains large amounts of sucrose and is generally to be used only in great moderation. Honey must be avoided by people with reactive hypoglycaemia, but there is some evidence that honey comb can afford protection against the ravages of hay fever (see page 98).

People who have been accustomed to taking large amounts of sugar and coffee or other refined foods sometimes find that, when they change to more natural high-fibre foods, they get odd days of exhaustion and depression. This may be because their digestion has difficulty in processing energy from these slow release foods after years of instant poor quality nourishment. A little honey may be an acceptable source of immediate energy to their exhausted digestive systems when combined with some protein source in, for example, an eggnog (see page 78).

Brown sugar. The only advantage that brown sugar has over white is that it is slightly less refined and, therefore, contains higher quantities of minerals and trace elements. *Molasses* is a further stage back in the refinement process and is quite rich in potassium and phosphorus. Both molasses and brown sugar, however, have the same physiological effect and they aggravate hypoglycaemia.

Sugar substitutes and artificial sweeteners are not to be recommended. Many of them are made from chemicals which are believed to irritate certain tissues of the body and may in time contribute to diseases such as cancer.

Coffee, tea, and the caffeine problem

There are various chemicals in coffee that may be a burden to your body but the principal trouble maker is caffeine, which also occurs to a lesser extent in tea, chocolate beverages, and cola drinks.

According to Doctors Stephen Davies and Alan Stewart, in *Nutritional Medicine* (Pan, 1987), as little as 50mg of caffeine can produce pharmacological effects. This is the amount contained in an average cup of strong tea, whilst a cup of coffee may contain 100mg.

Caffeine is a stimulant and prevents proper sleep in some people, but it can also depress the immune system. Caffeine reduces the amount of iron and zinc which is absorbed, especially when taken with meals, and it aggravates the low blood sugar syndrome. Given these facts, together with the usual practice of taking sugar with them, coffee and strong tea on a regular basis are clearly unsuitable for the hay fever sufferer.

Decaffeinated coffee may still contain a small percentage of caffeine and other chemicals which may be harmful, including those which have been used for the decaffeination process! Pleasant alternatives abound — see the Basic Diet and the recommendations which follow it.

Healthy combinations

According to Dr W.H. Hay, certain classes of food are not compatible when eaten together. They are inadequately digested and the chemical imbalance this causes may contribute to a wide variety of health problems. Dr Hay, whose system became known as the Hay Diet, maintained that sufferers from hay fever (no relation!) could, by his recommendations, expose themselves to pollens with impunity.

The Hay concept is based on the principle that the presence of starch or sugar with protein food neutralizes the acid medium required for protein digestion. The incomplete protein digestion results in larger molecules which cause allergy. Protein combined with a starch meal induces the secretion of more stomach acid which arrests the digestion of starches and sugars requiring an alkaline medium in the duodenum.

Our Basic Diet is not constructed strictly according to Hay principles. It is more important to introduce the essentials of wholefood eating first but, when you have, you may find that you can reduce your body's burden of irritants still further by avoiding 'foods that fight'. You will find a comprehensive description of the Hay System, with menus and recipes, in *Food Combining for Health* by Doris Grant and Jean Joice (Thorsons, 1984). The essentials are that obviously starchy or sugary foods, such as bread, potatoes, or puddings, should not be eaten with proteins (meat, eggs, nuts) and acid fruits (oranges, apples, grapefruits) in the same meal. Four hours should lapse between meals containing the different food groups.

A basic health diet

The suggestions given here are based on the general principles which have been discussed so far. I have outlined a wholefood menu adequate to maintain good health, low in fats, refined carbohydrates, and salt, and virtually free of the items which are likely to aggravate your hay fever.

A number of alternatives are given for each meal so that you can select to suit your taste and provide variety through the week. If you are not accustomed to this type of food don't be too daunted. Introduce these measures a little at a time, perhaps by changing the pattern of one meal, such as breakfast, for a week or two, before tackling the others.

But do start on this programme straight away even if the hay fever season is some way off. It takes time to change the body physiology and build up a better level of health and, no matter how bad or mild your symptoms, you will soon feel the general benefit.

BASIC HEALTH DIET

Daily Menu

On rising	Cider vinegar or lemon juice drink: one dessertspoonful in a cup of warm water with half a teaspoonful of honey if necessary. Fresh fruit juice or a herb tea may be used as an alternative.
Breakfast	One of the following may be taken. Fresh fruit in season, dried fruit (e.g., apricots, prunes), baked or puréed apple with raisins, muesli, wholemeal or rye bread toasted or fresh, with unsalted butter or sunflower margarine and honey, pure fruit jam, or savoury spread. If a drink is required, a glass of pure unsweetened fruit juice, China or herb tea, coffee substitute, or other hot drink as described on page 58 may be taken.
Mid-morning	If a drink is required, choose from the list on page 58. If a snack is required use a wholemeal biscuit or a little fruit, nuts, or sunflower seeds.
Midday meal	Mixed vegetable salad containing the ingredients as described below with a baked jacket potato

and/or baked onion, and cheese or milled nuts. Salad dressing as described below. Wholemeal or rye bread or wholemeal biscuits with savoury spread.

or

Warm savoury dish (egg, lean meat, cheese, or nut or other savoury) with conservatively cooked vegetables and baked jacket potato, or cereal grains (see below). For dessert — soaked dried fruit, baked apple, fresh fruit, muesli, yogurt, soured milk, carrageen or natural fruit jelly.

Mid-afternoon	As mid-morning.
Evening meal	Alternative to midday meal. The salad meal may be taken at midday or in the evening according to preference and convenience. It is desirable to have one raw salad meal per day throughout the year. Dessert — as for lunch.
Before retiring	If a drink is required choose from the list on page 58. It is preferable not to eat unless you have low blood sugar problems.

HEALTHY FOOD PREPARATION

Salads

These must be fresh — not tinned or frozen. One meal a day should be a salad. Use as much variation as possible from the following ingredients:

Lettuce, tomatoes, Chinese leaves, mustard and cress, celery, red or white cabbage, carrots, radishes, cucumber, onions, beetroot (preferably raw and grated), watercress, chicory, garlic, endive, raisins, cottage or goat's milk cheese and milled nuts.

Salad dressing

This may consist of any mixture of oil (e.g., olive, sunflower, or corn oils), cider vinegar, dried skimmed milk, yogurt, soured milk, honey, lemon juice, herbs, garlic, and a pinch of sea salt to flavour. A suitable proportion is 75 per cent of oil mixed with 25 per cent cider vinegar or lemon juice and other constituents. No proprietary salad dressing should be used.

Meat

Use lean meats only. Meats should be grilled or baked. When baking, allow all fat to drain away. It is preferable to use only vegetable oil for cooking. Herbs and garlic may be added after cooking for flavouring.

Fish

This should be baked, grilled, or steamed — no fat to be used. Add herbs to flavour.

Eggs

These should be free-range whenever possible. They should not be eaten more than 3 or 4 times per week.

Other proteins

Vary the protein intake by using nuts, pulses (lentils, peas, beans, soya beans, and soya flour), grains, and seeds (sesame and sunflower seeds). Tofu (bean curd) is an excellent and versatile source of protein. Many recipes are to be found in vegetarian cookery books available from health food stores. Most pulses will require soaking for 24 hours before use.

Grains

These may be used as the main dish in place of other proteins. Use buckwheat, whole wheat, flaked or whole millet, brown rice, or flaked rice. Try to obtain organically grown grains. Packaged millet with a little cheese is available for easy preparation. Many stores now supply grains and pulses in larger quantities which reduces cost.

Cooking the grains

Place the grains in a saucepan and cover with water. Bring to the boil, replace the lid and allow to simmer for 5-10 minutes, when the grains should have absorbed most of the water. Add grated cheese, mushrooms, onions, cottage and/or curd cheese to flavour. Serve with vegetables or salad.

Sprouted grains and seeds

Uncooked sprouted grains are a highly nutritious addition to the diet which can be used in sandwiches or on salads. Sprouting trays are available from health food stores and some hardware stores. You can also spread the grains on moist blotting paper in a large dish or tray. Moisten each day with fresh water. Most grains will germinate within 2-3 days and may be eaten when the sprouts are half to one inch in length. Wheat, alfalfa, and sesame seeds are the most suitable for sprouting.

Vegetables

These should always be fresh. It is better to buy small quantities often. Whenever possible obtain organically grown, unsprayed vegetables. Use only conservative cooking methods and do not add salt.

Conservative cooking

Use for all vegetables and fruit. After preparation, place the vegetable, or fruit, in a saucepan and add 1-2 inches of water in the bottom, it is not necessary to cover them. Place the lid on the saucepan and bring to the boil and allow to simmer, adding more water if necessary. Cook until just tender and still slightly crisp. This method of cooking minimizes the loss of vitamins and minerals and retains the maximum flavour of the vegetable or fruit. Keep the water used in cooking for sauce or gravy stock.

Drinks

Strong coffee and Indian tea should be avoided. Use China tea or a good quality decaffeinated coffee or a coffee substitute, such as dandelion coffee or a good quality beverage made from barley, figs, and chicory which is available from health food stores.

Warm drinks can be made with low-sodium savoury extracts — one teaspoonful to a cup of hot water. Cider vinegar or lemon juice can be made into a drink, a teaspoon or dessertspoon of either ingredient is used in hot water according to taste. Another combination is lemon and honey.

Fruit juices should be fresh whenever possible. Tinned juices may be used but these should be unsweetened and free from additives or colouring. Bottled or tinned pineapple, grape, or apple juices may be used. Never use soft drinks, squashes, glucose drinks, colas, etc.

Vegetable juices are an excellent way of increasing vitamin and mineral intake. Use organically grown vegetables in a juice extractor either singly or mixed together. The lacto-fermented vegetable juices are particularly recommended. These contain bacteria closely resembling those found in the normal human intestine and which are necessary to good digestive function.

Alcohol

Should be kept to an absolute minimum. If taken regularly, spirits can prove harmful to the liver and kidneys, whilst beer depletes the body's vitamin B reserves as well as disturbing the blood sugar levels. Least harmful are the light table wines, but in normal health, other drinks are permissible on special occasions.

Microwave cooking

A microwave oven heats the food by increasing the rate of movement of its molecules. There is not yet enough evidence about the effects this has on the nutritional quality of the food but there is some loss of essential vitamins. If your diet contains plenty of fresh raw foods, and also traditionally cooked food, the occasional quick meal from a microwave will do no harm, but you should not rely on it for all your cooking.

Food irradiation

The practice of irradiating foods to kill pests and prolong shelf life is very controversial but is creeping in. It is not yet officially permitted in the U.K. It is argued that it does away with the need for chemical pesticides and preservatives, but it probably also does away with much of the biological value of the food as a source of high quality nutrition.

Buying wholefoods

It is not always easy to buy organically grown wholefoods. Create a demand by asking for these whenever possible. Certain shops, notably health food stores, specialize in some of the types of food referred to above. Grains and pulses can often be bought in bulk from special stores or a distribution network might have been set up in your area which offers a big saving. All bakers can supply wholemeal or wholewheat bread (specify this; not just 'brown bread'). Always insist on the correct product and do not be satisfied with substitutes.

5 Spring Clean Your Body

Special diets for hay fever relief

If you have managed to introduce some of my recommendations for healthier eating the probability is that you will be feeling generally better. Most people feel fitter in themselves, with more energy and improved skin complexion, even if their symptoms are still lurking. What you have done is to renovate your system's furnishings and polish the surfaces but, for all-through health, it needs a more thorough spring clean.

Once you can give your body an opportunity to dredge out the toxic residues which it stores away in the tissues — the chronic catarrh in sinuses and lungs, the devitalized and decaying cells in your sluggish skin, the overloaded lymphatics burdened by unresolved battles with past infections, and the fermenting waste by-passed in the corners of your colon — it will express its appreciation by becoming more effective at resisting the ravages of pollens and other allergens. Quite apart from the advantages in overcoming hay fever, you will be building an effective immunity against many other degenerative diseases. The causes of disease are fundamentally the same. It is its manifestations which vary.

Detoxifying programmes

In this chapter I shall give you some dietary detoxifying programmes. Their main benefits are felt by the stomach and intestines, but they will need to be supported by tonic measures to improve the function of other eliminative organs, such as the skin and lungs. Tonic sprays and friction rubs to improve skin function, and breathing exercises are described in later chapters. Herbs and homoeopathy will also play their part in the total programme of self-help.

Symptom aggravations

When vital functions have been suppressed — either by medical treatment, such as antibiotics and cold cures, or by eating excessively and inappropriately when suffering from infections — measures to rebuild your health may take you through a few aggravations of old symptoms.

These 'unfoldings' of old symptoms were defined by the pioneer naturopath, Dr Henry Lindlahr, as the 'healing crises'. The homoeopathic physician, Dr Hering, formulated the *Law of Cure* to describe the tendency for our bodies to go back through previously suppressed or unresolved acute symptoms, bringing to the surface what may have been driven deep by unsuitable treatment in the past.

The catarrhal child, whose repeated colds or earaches were suppressed with antibiotics, may, with a revision of diet and tonic measures described here, again experience some runny colds. The chronic catarrh lays the foundations for hay fever, but the well managed cold is our body's safety valve — let it take its course. The old saying about feeding a cold was really 'if you feed a cold you'll have to starve a fever'. In other words going on stuffing in starchy, clogging foods when the body is trying to get rid of impurities sometimes defeats its eliminative efforts and, although you may feel temporarily a little better, your body may eventually have to resort to strong measures, such as a feverish 'flu, to try to clear things.

Chronic respiratory troubles are often linked to skin problems, such as eczema, and if your hay fever has developed from an asthmatic background, particularly one in which infantile eczema was suppressed by creams or ointments, then don't be surprised to see some rashes reappearing.

These old symptoms are no cause for concern, and are certainly not a deterioration in your condition. In fact, most people report feeling better in themselves even though their symptoms are temporarily worse — a sure sign that their body is making a positive response.

Monitor your colon

Although you may have a regular bowel action

you might be surprised to learn that you can still be suffering from a form of constipation. Many people open their bowels daily but what they pass may be only at the front of the queue, so to speak, after taking several days to get there. It may also have left behind uneliminated faecal matter in pockets, known as diverticula, formed by distention of the weakened intestinal walls.

Normal transit time, the time it takes for food to be moved through the digestive tract and for its indigestible residue to be passed in stools, is about twelve hours. Some people's systems are so sluggish that it may take anything from 24 to 70 hours for food to pass through. This means that the rate of elimination of impurities from the blood and body tissues is correspondingly slowed down. When this happens, a lot of the fluid normally eliminated with the stools is reabsorbed causing waterlogging of the tissues and reducing the bulk of the stools. Healthy stools should be well formed, dark in colour and light enough to float.

Testing transit time

Before you undertake any cleansing diets it may be instructive to carry out a simple test of your transit time.

At about 9.00pm eat two charcoal biscuits, or swallow four charcoal tablets. You can obtain charcoal biscuits from your health food store, or the tablets from a chemist. The biscuits can be made palatable with some butter or margarine and a spread.

Observe your stools and note the time at which they first appear to be noticeably darkened or black. Then note when the black stools finally clear.

The healthy colon should clear everything in around twelve hours. This is all the time the efficient digestive system needs to cope with the various stages of breakdown of food and absorption of nutrients in the stomach and small intestines and for the residues to pass on to the colon for bacterial activity and collection of impurites from the body fluids. If your transit time is much longer than this there is likely to be a hold up somewhere, and your intestines may appreciate a pause in the downward pressure to enable them to clear some of the backlog. Fasting or cleansing diets will provide the needed rest and benefit other parts of your system as well.

How fasting helps hay fever

Witholding solid food is an ancient practice. From

earliest times man would instinctively stop eating when he felt unwell; wild animals still do. Feverish children lose their appetites and should not be encouraged to eat. Hay fever sufferers can gain great relief by doing the same.

Witholding solid food and fasting on raw fruit and vegetable juices has proven physiological benefits. Here are just some of the advantages that the hay fever sufferer will derive from fasting:

- Resting the digestive functions enables the body to direct energy to the healing of inflamed surfaces.

- The high alkalinity of raw juices counteracts tissue acidity and reduces the irritation of mucous surfaces.

- Raw juices are rich in vitamins and minerals required for your body's immunity and detoxifying processes.

- The level of heat due to feverish activity in the nose and sinuses will be reduced.

- The elimination of decaying unhealthy cells is speeded up.

- The regeneration of new healthy cells is increased.

- The lymphatic system, cleared of debris, is able to function more efficiently in its task of filtering impurities and maintaining body defence.

- After fasting the rested digestive system can work with increased efficiency to provide good quality nourishment for the process of regeneration.

The membranes of nose and sinuses in the hay fever victim become like a battlefield awash with histamine, and the spent and exhausted mast cells and lymphocytes are more effectively cleared and eliminated by fasting.

Choosing the intensity of treatment

Cleansing diets can be of varying intensity. Fasting will be the strictest, but the most effective, whilst raw fruit or vegetable diets rank a little lower in efficiency. The vital component or 'sunlight value' of raw juices and fruits encourages the cleansing activity and this would, therefore, be less efficient in cooked vegetables and with the introduction of starches, such as rice or wholemeal bread. The elimination will be slower in such cases. The grades of cleansing diet are:

> Fasting — water only
> Raw juice diet
> Raw fruit diet
> Mono diet — fruit or cereals only
> Raw fruit and vegetables
> Cooked fruit and vegetables
> Wholefood vegetarian diet
> Wholefood mixed diet

The stricter the diet the more the relief to the hay fever sufferer since the reduction of inflammation and catarrhal congestion is likely to be speeded up. It may not always be convenient, however, for you to follow stricter phases of the cleansing programme, but your hay fever will still be relieved by undertaking the less stringent measures of, for example, a raw fruit and vegetable diet.

The fasts and diets described here are good ways of reducing the susceptibility to hay fever and rhinitis and can also be applied for the relief of the acute symptoms. Try these in the weeks preceding the pollen plague but, for more alleviation of the acute allergic manifestations, you could attempt the *Fast Relief Plan* which incorporates other measures and supportive supplements. The Fast Relief Plan is described fully on page 171.

After a conventional diet of meat, dairy produce, sugar, salt, and refined flour, even the adoption of the Basic Diet will have a moderately cleansing and rejuvenating effect.

Break yourself in gradually

If you have never fasted or eaten a lot of fresh raw fruit or vegetables you may find it easier to introduce yourself gradually to the cleansing programme. This may be particularly necessary if your hay fever is superimposed on a chronic background of asthma, eczema, and other allergic disorders. You will certainly derive more benefit from extended cleansing programmes but should introduce them slowly or under the supervision of a qualified naturopath or a doctor who is experienced in the management of fasts.

Children from the ages of 3-4 years can, on the other hand, be fasted more readily and, because of their quicker metabolism, will respond quite dramatically.

If you have adopted the general scheme of the basic diet you can break yourself in over a period of a few weeks by introducing one day a week on raw foods only. Then, when you feel ready, you can make it a fruit and juices day once a week followed, say once a fortnight, by the fruit and salads day.

What to expect with fasts and light diets

When you undertake a juice fast, or a few days on raw food or fruit, you may become aware of some sensations which indicate that your body is beginning the process of detoxification. There may be some hunger and rumbles from your stomach and intestines. Don't worry; they are just due to the slight fermentation which accompanies the digestion of extra cellulose and fibrous material.

You may experience a slight headache on the first day or two and the tongue may become dry and coated. The breath may smell unpleasant and there may be a metallic or bitter taste in the mouth. There will be an increased output of urine and it may become darker as it carries more impurities. The bowels may become looser, perhaps with a little diarrhoea (although if there isn't much bowel activity when you are on the juices only diet an enema may be necessary). The skin elimination will increase and perspiration may become more odorous for a while. (Don't use roll-on anti-perspirants — they shut off the pores and depress the natural skin function.)

All these are beneficial responses which generally clear after two or three days but, best of all for the hay fever case, there will be an increase in elimination of old catarrh, a gradual clearing of the nasal and sinus congestion, and a renewed ease of breathing with a reduction of the itching and burning sensation of the eyes and throat.

Cleansing menus

Here are suggested menus for these introductory cleansing routines.

Raw food day

On rising	One dessertspoonful of lemon juice or apple cider vinegar with a little honey in a mug of warm water or herb tea (e.g. chamomile, peppermint, or rose hip).
Breakfast	Fresh raw fruit, e.g. apples, pears, grapes, oranges, pineapple, peaches, or melon. Eat sufficient to satisfy appetite.
Mid-morning	Herb tea or freshly extracted fruit juice or canned or bottled unsweetened juice or mineral water with a slice of lemon. If hungry an apple or a pear may be eaten.
Lunch	A small glass of freshly extracted or bottled lacto-fermented vegetable or fruit juice (e.g., carrot, celery, beetroot), or combined fruit and vegetable juices available in cans.
	Mixed vegetable salad containing a selection of vegetables as recommended on page 56 and garnished with herbs. Salad dressing (see page 57).
Afternoon	As mid-morning.
Evening meal	As for lunch or mixed fruit salad with a few sunflower or pumpkin seeds scattered over it. Add a little almond cream or runny honey to flavour.
On retiring	Herb tea or savoury extract drink.

A fresh fruit day

On rising	One dessertspoonful of lemon juice or apple cider vinegar in warm water (add a little honey to taste), or fresh fruit juice or herb tea.

Main meals	Each meal may consist of a selection of fresh fruit in season. Eat sufficient to satisfy the appetite. Choose from: apples, pears, grapes, oranges, pineapples, paw paw, passion fruit, peaches, melons, or other fruit in season (except bananas which are too starchy). Fruits can be eaten singly or chopped or grated to form a fruit salad over which a little honey or maple syrup may be poured. If you keep to one type of fruit, such as grapes, the detoxifying effect tends to be greater.
Between meals	Drink mineral water with a slice of lemon or a pure freshly extracted or bottled or canned unsweetened juice. If you want a warm drink use concentrated pure apple juice with hot water or cider vinegar and honey.
On retiring	Herb tea or fruit juice as above.

How and when to fast

If you have managed a fresh fruit day once a week for several weeks with success you may feel able to embark upon a short fast. In fact, if you are experiencing acute hay fever symptoms this would be an excellent way of relieving them. It will also be a good rehearsal for the Fast Relief Plan which is a more intensive programme for coping with bad symptoms.

The juice fast can be undertaken for from one to three days or longer. There are many cases on record of people who have fasted for 40 to 80 days, remaining vigorous and active throughout. Longer fasts, however, should not be undertaken without some professional supervision. The longer you fast the more gradual should be your return to a normal diet.

The following plan for a 24 hour fast can be extended to several days if you feel well on it. It may be wise to begin at a weekend when you have less to do physically, but it is usually better to remain reasonably active or do some gentle exercise, like walking in the fresh air, to promote the functions of lungs and skin.

The juice fast

(This fast may be followed for 1-5 days)

On rising	One glass of hot water with the juice of half a lemon or one dessertspoonful of lemon juice or apple cider vinegar.
Breakfast	One large tumbler of freshly expressed juice of either apple, grape, carrot, orange, or pineapple. These may be diluted with a little mineral water. Canned or bottled juices may be used but must be pure, unsweetened, and free from preservatives or other additives (if using pineapple juice dilute it by half with mineral water).
Mid-morning	One glass of mineral water with a slice of lemon.
Lunch	Pure juice as for breakfast. You may combine two juices, such as carrot and apple or orange and pineapple.
Mid-afternoon	One glass of mineral water with a slice of lemon.
Evening	Pure juices either singly or combined, as for lunch.
On retiring	Warm water with one teaspoonful of vegetable concentrate or yeast extract or concentrated apple juice.

How to break the fast

You can undo the benefits of the fast or cleansing diet if you reintroduce normal food too quickly. Remember you will have set in motion the detoxifying mechanisms of the body and these will need to continue gently for several days after the initial stimulus of the physiological rest from solid food. After a fast of two or three days the mucous membranes of the nose and sinuses may begin to mobilize old congestive catarrhal deposits which are a focus for further infections and perpetuate the susceptibility to pollinosis. Introducing the wrong sorts of foods too soon could abort this cleansing process.

Ideally, the 24 hour fast should be followed by either a raw food or fruit day, with, if something warm is desired, the potassium broth (see page 175). If you have fasted for several days then the reintroduction of food should be made gradually, building up with vitalizing nutrients.

The Transition Diet should follow fasts of three or more days but is helpful after any stricter programme.

Transition diet

First day

Fruit juice or hot water and lemon drink on rising.

For breakfast eat a finely grated raw apple or some grapes. Continue with the juices but add a small mixed salad for lunch (coarse ingredients should be grated or finely chopped).

In the evening have fresh fruit again, such as grapes, melons, paw paw, or peaches.

Second day

(Recommence any supplements or herbal medicines you may be taking.) Continue the fruit juices as before.

Fresh or soaked dried fruit (e.g. prunes, apricots) and a small container of plain goat's milk yogurt.

For lunch a small mixed salad with a little dried fruit and milled nuts and salad dressing (see page 56). Fresh fruit to follow.

Dinner may be a salad as for lunch or a mixed vegetable stew.

Third day

As for the second day, but you may add some seeds or nuts to the breakfast; savoury rice portion or baked jacket potato with sunflower margarine with the salad meal; a slice of wholemeal bread with margarine and savoury spread with the stew in the evening. Use juices as before between the meals or lacto-fermented bottled vegetable juices as an aperitif to the main meals.

Fourth day onwards

After this, return to the full Basic Diet, but be prepared for mild symptoms or aggravations — quite normal as the eliminative process continues.

You should endeavour to eat slowly and chew your food well.

FULL SCALE SPRING CLEAN DIET

This is an extended but easy to follow cleansing programme, ideal for the early spring, prior to the onset of the hay fever season. It will reduce the toxic load and clear out residual catarrh from winter colds and 'flu. You can, of course, do this spring-clean programme at any time of the year.

Spring Clean Programme

First three days

Commence the treatment with three days on fresh fruit and/or vegetable juices only. (Try 24 hours on juices and two days on fruit.) If on juices, take one tumblerful 4-5 times per day. You may take as much as your appetite demands of any fresh fruit. Any kind of fresh fruit, except rhubarb and bananas, may be taken. If you have rheumatism or arthritis or skin problems you should also avoid citrus fruit. No sugar, either white or brown, must be used for sweetening. If any fruit cannot be eaten without sweetening omit it.

Drinks during this first three days should consist of pure unsweetened fruit or vegetable juices, e.g., apple, grape, (orange), pineapple (dilute 50 per cent). If a warm drink is required you may have one teaspoonful of vegetable extract (available from a health food store) dissolved in a cup of hot water. Mineral water or plain water is permissible.

On the second day a small warm water enema should be taken (see instructions on page 107). If there is normal bowel action on the second morning the enema may not be necessary, but is nevertheless a valuable cleansing measure.

Fourth to seventh days

Breakfast

Drink of fruit juice. Fresh fruit as desired or baked apple with raisins (see page 179).

Between meals	Herb teas, fruit juice, or savoury extract in warm water.
Lunch	Raw salad with dressing as described on page 56. As a dessert use fresh fruit only, cut up into fruit salad sprinkled with wheat germ or milled nuts, and moistened with unsweetened pineapple or grape juice, if desired.
Evening meals	Raw salad again and dressing, or vegetable broth flavoured with vegetable or yeast extract. For dessert, use fresh fruit or baked or stewed apple or soaked dried prunes or apricots.

Second week

Breakfast	Fresh fruit or baked or stewed apple or dried fruit (e.g., raisins, apricots, prunes). Nuts if desired with the fruit. A fruit salad may be made with wheat germ or grated nuts sprinkled over it and a syrup of honey and water to flavour.
Between meals	Herb tea, savoury drink, or fruit juice. Juices may be taken as an aperitif to main meals.
Lunch	Raw salad as before or the mid-day meal and evening meal may be transposed. Raisins or sultanas or a few whole or grated nuts may be added to the salad to give variety. You may also have one or two slices of brown rye bread or rye biscuits with a scraping of butter and a small portion of low fat cheese with the salad. Alternatively, a baked jacket potato, with a little sunflower seed oil. Fresh fruit as dessert.
Evening meal	Two or three conservatively cooked vegetables. Light savoury dish made with eggs, low fat cheese, nuts, tofu, or cereal grains (e.g., brown rice, millet, buckwheat, or rye). Steamed fish may be used as an alternative, or vegetable broth or stew. Fresh fruit as dessert.

If the juice and fruit days are not possible or convenient you may do a modified version of this diet by starting at the fourth day and continuing from there with the rest of the two week programme.

Some cautions for diets and fasting

Most people can undertake these cleansing diets without harm, but there are a few situations in which fasting may not be suitable.

If, when you miss a meal, you experience weakness, dizziness, detachment, or headaches, you may have functional hypoglycaemia. In which case juice or water fasts would not be suitable but you could try fruit days. Take a little fruit every three or four hours rather than just at normal meal times.

People with serious disorders, such as cancer, TB, diabetes, or heart disease, should not undertake fasts without medical guidance. They will, of course, derive great benefit from the Basic Diet, to build up vitality and reduce their toxic burden. Caution should be observed with infants and very small children as well as the elderly and frail. They can usually cope with modifications to the diet such as the introduction of more vegetables and fruit, in an easily digestible form, and the reduction of the mucous forming foods.

Fortunately, fasting and dietetic treatments are safe and extremely effective regenerative procedures for most of us throughout our active lives.

Supplementary measures

Although dietetic management and the cleansing programmes are at the core of your treatment to eradicate hay fever, there are other important measures to encourage elimination from skin, lungs, bowels, and kidneys.

The American naturopath and nutritionist, Paavo Airola, attached great importance to the use of the enema during fasting. He found that patients undergoing juice fasts in his clinic got more effective elimination without the unpleasant feelings associated with the mobilization of toxins and their release into the blood stream. I have also found that my patients make a speedier recovery from acute feverish conditions, especially those of the respiratory system, when a small enema is used in conjunction with a fast.

It is important, however, that enemas, and the more extended form of bowel cleansing, colonic irrigation, should only be used when you are actually fasting. They should not become a substitute for regular and natural bowel function. If the bowels are sluggish and weak it would be better to use a gentle bulk action herbal laxative whilst eating. Full instructions for the use of the enema are given in Chapter 9.

Lung function is increased by breathing exercises and physical activity such as brisk walking. Regular walking in the open air, while undergoing the spring clean programmes, ensures good lung function and exposure to natural daylight, which is important for the body's internal equilibrium. It is especially helpful to take advantage of the fresh air and sunlight before the pollens become problematic.

The rigours of diets and fasts are not the only way to hay fever relief. Nature has provided other aids to better function in the form of herbs and homoeopathic medicines which can back up the benefits of the cleansing programmes, and the vital regenerative phases can be supported with suitable vitamin and mineral supplements.

6 *Putting the Power in Nutrition*

The role of vitamins and minerals

The science of nutrition has made enormous strides in the last fifty years. More and more is being discovered about the vital role of vitamins, minerals, trace elements, amino acids, and essential fatty acids in our body economy and yet, what we know may only be the tip of the iceberg of our bodies' complex biochemical processes. Even in this age of sophisticated scientific technology the wisdom of nature, which has stood us in good stead over several million years, is unlikely to be revealed in its entirety for a very long time, if ever.

Nevertheless, with the knowledge at our disposal we know that it is possible and necessary to potentiate the power of what may be considered to be good basic nutrition. Not much more than fifty years ago we knew little or nothing of the vitamins, the role of the trace elements had not been thought about, and no one had heard about essential fatty acids, yet mankind survived — on the whole with less degenerative disease and certainly fewer allergies.

The need for nutritional supplements

So why should we need nutritional supplements? The cynics will argue that the average diet contains adequate nutrients to meet recommended dietary allowances (RDAs). They are basing their views on chemical simplicity and not on biological reality. The RDAs are average figures based on minimal amounts needed to overcome

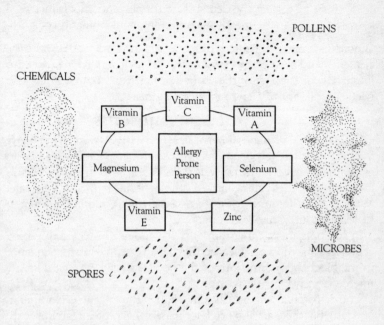

Figure 6. Front-line nutrients.

obvious deficiencies. They take no account of our individuality, both genetically and biochemically, which can make our nutritional needs very much greater, especially under additional stress or threat by invaders, such as pollens.

Even with the higher nutritional quality of the Basic Diet described here you may fall short of your body's requirements for adequate energy production and immune competence. The reasons for this are:

- modern farming methods, as we have already seen, result in soil mineral deficiencies;

- chemical residues from farming and food processing interfere with cellular activity, and reduce the levels of essential nutrients;

- declining vitality and insidious deficiency impairs the digestive functions, reducing absorption of vital nutrients from food;

- the demand for certain nutrients is increased greatly in conditions of inflammation or stress.

Wholefoods are rich sources of many vitamins, minerals, and trace elements, and by selective eating of the foods richest in them you can improve your supplies of the 'front-line nutrients', but you may also need to use naturally prepared supplements.

Front-line nutrients

Certain vitamins and minerals are particularly important for hay fever sufferers because of the vital role they play in either the function of the mucous membranes, or in the body defence mechanisms. These are what I call the *front-line nutrients*. They are: Vitamin A; Vitamin B complex, especially B_6; Vitamin C; Vitamin E; Magnesium; Zinc; Selenium.

In addition, many other nutrients play indirect or supportive roles, acting in some cases as synergists (having an essential interdependence in the biochemical functions of the body, e.g., zinc and calcium are interdependent).

The *support nutrients* are calcium, vitamin P, manganese, chromium, and iron, but there are also needs for many other proteins (amino acids) and essential fatty acids (EFAs). They are important because of their function in maintaining general bodily health rather than any direct involvement in the prevention of hay fever, although the EFAs, for example, do play an important role in prostaglandin synthesis.

MINERALS

Probably the most important nutrients are the minerals. They are the basic chemicals of life. All living matter is composed of the elements carbon, hydrogen, oxygen, and nitrogen. The major structural and physiological minerals are calcium, magnesium, phosphorus, potassium, sodium, and chlorine. In addition, we require small daily amounts of the trace elements, iron, zinc, copper, manganese, iodine, chromium, and selenium.

According to Dr Leslie H. Fisher, of the International Mineral Therapy Association, correct mineral metabolism is a basic prerequisite to healthy nutrition. When our mineral needs are met in the biologically available form we tend to utilize other nutrients from our food with greater efficiency.

Mineral supplements
Minerals are active in our bodies in a compound form. A positive ion (cation) unites with a negative ion (anion); for example, the cation magnesium combines with the anion phosphorus to form magnesium phosphate. In this form they are carried to the cell membrane where it can absorb its requirements selectively.

Some authorities believe that more active absorption from the intestines, and by the individual cells of the body, is possible when the mineral is combined with an organic compound, such as orotic acid, or an amino acid chelate (chelation is the process of binding of a mineral to a protein compound). You will find most mineral supplements are now sold as the orotate or the chelate which is a good form to ensure absorption, though many naturopaths prefer the physiologically less crude approach of the Celloid formulations, in which the mineral compounds are prescribed in physiological doses according to the patient's individual health indications.

Choosing supplements
So many supplements are now sold, either singly or in compounds, and the choice may seem a nightmare. Be guided by your health food store proprietor who will usually stock the best brands. Health food stores may also have combined vitamin, mineral, and herbal formulations suitable for hay fever and rhinitis.

Dosage of mineral supplements
Unless specifically recommended, dosage will vary according to the strength and form in which a particular mineral is available. Be guided by the manufacturer's recommendations unless more specific figures are given in the descriptions which follow.

Magnesium
Magnesium is a catalyst (initiates change) in many chemical reactions of the body. It has close links with calcium, especially in the movement of minerals across the cell membrane. It is, therefore, an important stabilizer of the mast cells, preventing the influx of calcium, which reacts with the IgE to trigger histamine release.

Magnesium is also important in carbohydrate metabolism, as it helps to buffer against the hyperinsulinism which lowers the blood sugar level.

Sources	Magnesium is found especially in nuts, seafoods, soya beans, grains, green leafy vegetables (in which it is a component of chlorophyll), and hard water.
Synergists	Vitamins B_1, B_6, calcium. The calcium to magnesium ratio should be 2:1 in the body. (Cow's milk is low in magnesium and high in calcium, so children who take a lot of milk become deficient in magnesium.)
Supplements	Magnesium orotate, magnesium amino chelate, Celloid magnesium phosphate. Normal daily requirement 350mg.

Calcium

Almost all of the total body calcium is required for the bones and teeth. Only about one per cent, in solution, is concerned with biochemical functions, but it is a very important one per cent. Calcium is readily lost in sweat, urine, and faeces, and mothers often worry about replacing it when they take their children off cow's milk for their catarrh and hay fever. As you will see from the list of sources there are plenty of alternative calcium-rich foods.

Dr Carl Pfeiffer, of the Brain Bio Center in Princeton, New Jersey, has found that 500mg of calcium gluconate, taken morning and evening, reduces the blood histamine of patients whose level is normally rather high, such as hypoglycaemics. Calcium ions promote histamine release but the calcium binds to the amino acid methionine to prevent this occurring.

Sources	Legumes, green leafy vegetables, broccoli, nuts, seeds, soya milk, and egg shells! (Dr Pfeiffer, in his book *Mental and Elemental Nutrients*, suggests standing an egg in cider vinegar for 24 hours to soften the shell and then using the whole egg, with shell, in a blender to make an eggnog.)
Synergists	Magnesium, zinc.
Supplements	Calcium orotate, or gluconate, or amino chelate. Also in dolomite (with magnesium, but ensure that this is a brand free of toxic metals such as lead and

mercury), and bone meal. Calcium needs efficient stomach acids for adequate absorption.

Potassium

This is another essential mineral for glucose metabolism. It is necessary at various stages of the energy cycle and is particularly important for the nervous system. Potassium sulphate is active in the transport system across cell membranes and can be helpful to promote better drainage of excess mucous from congested nose and sinuses.

Sources	Fruit (especially grapes), vegetables, root vegetables (save and use the liquid in which they are cooked), wheat germ, lentils, nuts.
Synergists	Magnesium, sodium.
Supplements	A physiologically balanced compound of potassium is preferable (e.g. Celloid potassium phosphate or potassium sulphate). It is also available as an orotate and chelate.

Sodium

Sodium is mentioned here largely because people take too much salt in food. This causes a relative deficiency of potassium and magnesium, and excess sodium can lead to fluid retention and catarrhs. Natural sodium is important in the body and in physiological or homoeopathic doses the compound sodium sulphate can promote the movement of fluids and the release of catarrhal deposits.

There is seldom any need to supplement sodium. You should get all you need from vegetables and grains in your diet.

TRACE ELEMENTS

Iron

Iron is an important part of many enzyme systems and, although it may be deficient in anaemic conditions, there is a greater danger in overdosing through self-prescribing of iron supplements. Too much iron depresses the levels of zinc, for example.

It is better to use a biochemic or homoeopathic form of iron to raise the body's level in anaemic states.

Sources   Organ meats, egg yolks, legumes, shellfish, parsley, watercress, green peppers.

Zinc

Zinc is a vital but vulnerable trace element. It is often removed in food processing, is antagonized in the body by copper and iron supplements, and its absorption is reduced by coffee, cow's milk, lemon, wholemeal bread, and bran. Zinc is vital to our growth and development and especially to our immune competence. It is important in maintaining glucose tolerance and in the metabolism of essential fatty acids.

Sources   Wholewheat, rye, oats, soya lecithin, muscle meats, Brazil nuts, egg yolk, almonds, walnuts, buckwheat, garlic, and potatoes.

Synergists   Zinc works in tandem with chromium in the maintenance of good sugar metabolism and also requires vitamin B_6 and vitamin C in many of the body chemistry changes with which it is involved.

Supplements   Zinc orotate, zinc gluconate. According to Drs Stephen Davis and Alan Stewart, in *Nutritional Medicine* (Pan, 1987), zinc supplements are better absorbed if taken at night when other nutrients will not interfere with them.

Copper

The levels of copper tend to rise during the premenstrual phase in women and this may antagonize zinc in the body. Copper is, nevertheless, important to some enzyme functions and actual deficiency of copper has been found to impair the immunity.

Sources   Liver, legumes, nuts.

Supplements   Copper is found in small amounts in multi-mineral supplements and is unlikely to be necessary for the hay fever sufferer in any other form apart from foods in which it occurs naturally.

Chromium

Chromium is known as the 'glucose tolerance factor' because it combines with B vitamins and amino acids to assist in the regulation of blood sugar levels.

Sources	Brewer's yeast (especially for the glucose tolerance factor), black pepper, wheat germ, wholemeal bread, brown rice, walnuts.
Synergists	Vitamin B_3, amino acids, zinc.
Supplements	Brewer's yeast.

Manganese

Manganese also plays a role in carbohydrate and protein metabolism. It activates enzymes necessary for the utilization of vitamin C and vitamins of the B complex.

Sources	Leafy vegetables, whole grains, tea (1mg/cup).
Supplements	10-20 milligrams per day of manganese chloride or manganese amino chelate. (Don't try to drink 10-20 cups of tea per day!)

Selenium

Selenium has recently assumed importance as a vital body protector. It reduces oxidation and, therefore, protects us against the action of free radicals which lower the vitality of cellular function.

Sources	Brewer's yeast, garlic, liver, eggs.
Synergists	Vitamin E.
Supplements	Functions with vitamin E. A good combination of selenium with vitamins A, C and E is available from health food stores.

Toxic metals

Some trace elements are harmful to the body when they enter it in too great a quantity. They may be consumed with our food, absorbed through the skin, or inhaled with polluted air. Although natural supplements of selenium with vitamin E are protective against the toxic metals, too much selenium in the form in which it is presented in some anti-dandruff shampoos may be harmful to the body when absorbed through the skin. (It is better to prevent dandruff by restricting your intake of refined carbohydrates.)

Lead, mercury, and aluminium are known to interfere with enzymes in the body and to depress the immune system. Lettuce, cabbage, and other green vegetables which are displayed outside a greengrocer's shop on a busy road will pick up significant quantities of lead from the petrol fumes of passing vehicles. Aluminium utensils are a source of toxicity if vegetables and fruits are cooked in them regularly. The acid in the fruit acts on the aluminium surface to dissolve it, and it is taken up by the food. Aluminium also occurs in kitchen foil, antacids (indigestion medicines), and anti-perspirants.

Fortunately, many ingredients of the wholefood diet are protective against damage from the toxic metals. Other than avoiding exposure to them, which we should all do, only the very hypersensitive need take special supplements to neutralize toxic metals and this should be done with professional guidance.

VITAMINS

These are essential ingredients of our diet which affect every aspect of our bodily function, particularly the integrity of the mucous membranes and immune system. Vitamins are abundant in fresh fruit, vegetables, wholegrains, seeds, and nuts — the main components of the wholefood diet. They are deficient in refined and processed foods and, furthermore, there is evidence that many of the additives used in food processing interfere with the body's absorption of vitamins. Vitamins play important synergistic roles with many essential minerals.

Vitamin A

The stability of the mucous membranes is of paramount importance to the hay fever sufferer. Healthy well nourished membranes keep the pollens and other allergens at bay, and one of the essentials for healthy membranes is vitamin A. It is also protective of the skin, so may help if you have excessive sensitivity or eczema.

Vitamin A is a fat-soluble vitamin, which means that it is carried around the body and stored in fats, so it is better to use it in conjunction with supplements such as vitamin E. Like vitamin E and some trace elements it has anti-oxidant properties.

Sources	Fish, liver, kidneys, eggs, carrots, cabbage, oranges, and other yellow fruits.
Supplements	Vitamin A can be toxic in high doses taken over several months but up to 10,000 IU daily may be taken by most adults with complete safety. Children should use about 5,000 IU daily.
Synergists	Best used with vitamin E, vitamin C, and selenium.

Vitamin B

Vitamin B is a complex of related vitamins, a number of which are important to hay fever sufferers. They are all found in similar foods and most are interdependent; for example vitamin B_2 and vitamin B_6 work in tandem and B_6 is closely linked to zinc in body metabolism. They are all involved in sugar digestion, essential fatty acid metabolism, and anti-inflammatory mechanisms. It is nearly always best to supplement the whole complex.

Sources	Liver, organ meats, whole grains, brewer's yeast, eggs, green leafy vegetables.
Supplements	Brewer's yeast, B complex preparations (hypoallergenic formulations are best). Vitamin B_6 and folic acid may be necessary in addition, especially the latter in children on goat's milk. Make them eat their greens!

Vitamin C

Vitamin C is one of the most important nutrients to the hay fever sufferer. It is a powerful anti-oxidant preventing the breakdown of cell membranes and playing a vital role in immunity and in anti-inflammatory activity. The most ardent advocate of vitamin C is Dr Linus Pauling, the American Nobel Prize winner, who believes that mankind in eons past consumed a diet of seeds and berries which provided many more times the vitamin C than we get in the modern diet. He and other researchers have repeatedly demonstrated that, where levels have been low, supplementation of considerable quantities can speed up recovery from colds and other inflammatory conditions, though its preventive action is less well proven.

Vitamin C is water-soluble and, therefore, unstable and easily lost. We cannot make it from other foods so it must be provided in our diet. It almost always needs to be supplemented at times of stress, infections, and when you have hay fever. Smokers lose up to 25 milligrams with every cigarette and non-smokers in the same room will also suffer losses, so all these people need to replace it regularly.

Sources	Fruits, green leafy vegetables, broccoli, sprouts, cauliflower, liver, potatoes, green peppers.
Supplements	Should be taken in a combined form with bioflavonoids (vitamin P), with which the C is found in nature. Five hundred milligrams to one gram daily (but caution with long-term administration if you have a history of kidney stones or you are on the low-dose contraceptive pill).

Vitamin E

This is another fat-soluble vitamin with anti-oxidant properties. This means that it protects the cells against the damage of the free radicals from chemicals in foods. Vitamin E is necessary to prevent oxidation of polyunsaturated fats which leads to rancidity. If you consume polyunsaturated vegetable oils, for example, adequate vitamin E is necessary but, generally, it is naturally present in them and in good quality margarines.

Sources	Vegetable oils, wheat germ, soya products, lettuce, eggs, nuts, seeds.
Synergists	Vitamin C, vitamin A, selenium.
Supplements	Natural vitamin E 400-600 IU per day.

How helpful for hay fever?

It is difficult to say how helpful specific supplements are for hay fever. Our bodies use varying quantities of nutrients according to individual need, so one person may find vitamin C valuable whilst another may swear by zinc. The important thing is that supplements can only really be of value in the context of a complete programme of health promotion, especially a natural food diet.

How to take vitamins and minerals

It will be obvious from the sources of nutrients described here that the best way of providing them is in your wholefood diet. Supplements, however, can build up the levels of important nutrients in a quick and easily absorbed form.

Generally the best way of boosting your mineral intake is to use a natural multi-mineral supplement available from a health food store. Some are made up in combination with important vitamins. For more specific needs, especially during the hay fever season, recommendations are made below.

Make sure that the supplements you take are prepared from natural ingredients and not synthesized with chemical raw materials. Natural supplements are concentrated and made from the foods which contain them.

Do not use single supplements, such as vitamin C, like another drug. You will do your body a disservice since all nutrients have important interactions. Remember that the term 'supplement' means an adjunct or back-up to a healthy diet. It is not a substitute.

A supplement programme for hay fever

The table of nutritional supplements on page 86 has been designed to provide those which may be of particular benefit to the hay fever case. For more specific and individual needs you should consult a natural therapy practitioner.

AMINO ACIDS

Amino acids are the building blocks of proteins. There are a number of them which are essential to bodily functions but, because we cannot manufacture them from raw materials in our food, they must be provided in the diet. These are the Essential Amino Acids (EAAs). EAAs are provided by the first-class proteins such as meat, fish, eggs, and dairy products. Vegetable foods, as second-class

SUPPLEMENTS FOR HAY FEVER

Nutrient	Strength	Adult's dose	Child's dose	Comments
Vitamin A	5,000 IU	2-3 per day	1 daily	
Vitamin B complex		Usually 1 daily of a strong formulation		
Vitamin C	500 mg	2-4 per day	1-2 per day	use Bioflavonoids
Vitamin E	100 IU	3-6 per day	2 daily	start low dose with high blood pressure; caution on heart drugs
Magnesium orotate*	250 mg	2 daily	1 daily	may be combined in Dolomite, 2 tabs 3 times daily
Calcium orotate*	500 mg	2 daily	1 daily	
Potassium orotate*	150 mg	3 daily	1 daily	take with meals
Selenium orotate*	50 mcg	2 daily	1 daily	always with vit E
Zinc orotate*	50 mg	1 daily	1 daily	best at night

*The strength of these minerals and trace elements may vary by brand. In most cases they may be more conveniently taken as a mulit-mineral supplement or in other combinations, such as selenium with vitamins A, C, and E.

proteins, do not contain them all. Vegetarians can make up the EAAs by combining foods such as grains and pulses in a ratio of three to one.

All the EAAs are important to our health in some way, but the need for the hay fever sufferer to take specific supplements of them is not, at this stage, particularly strongly indicated. The Basic Diet provides all your requirements for amino acids, but there are two which are so important that the need to ensure supplies of them in the foods you eat cannot be overstressed.

Methionine is an anti-oxidant which combines with the free radicals which might damage cells in the body. It also plays an important role in detoxifying histamine in those whose blood levels are high, according to Dr C. Pfeiffer. Methionine combines with the calcium which would otherwise move into the mast cells with IgE to release histamine. Methionine is also necessary for the transport of selenium. Main food sources of methionine are chicken, beef, fish, cottage cheese, yogurt, sesame seeds, and lentils.

Glutathione is a compound of three amino acids, cysteine, glutamic acid, and glycine, which plays an important protective role in the immune system. It also assists the removal of toxic metals and free radicals from the body. Its presence in onions and garlic explains their value as detoxifiers.

ESSENTIAL FATTY ACIDS

Some fatty acids are, like the amino acids, essential to our metabolic functions and must be provided in our diet. Essential fatty acids (EFAs) help to transport the fat-soluble vitamins, such as vitamin A and vitamin E, and they are also important for the synthesis of the protective prostaglandin, PGE_1.

All the EFAs are polyunsaturated fats; that is to say they are liquid at room temperature, such as vegetable oils. The two most important ones are linolenic acid and linoleic acid. Gamma-linolenic acid (GLA) is present in human breast milk and also found in the Evening primrose plant.

Sources	Vegetable oil margarines, sunflower and safflower oils, leafy vegetables, nuts, and seeds.
Synergists	Vitamin B complex, vitamins C and E, zinc, and magnesium.
Supplements	Evening primrose oil (seeds contain 10 per cent GLA), fish oils.

7 Herbs and Homoeopathy

Safe and soothing support

Although we possess remarkable self-healing capabilities our bodies do need help from time to time, especially in the alleviation of acute symptoms such as those of hay fever. There are limits to the efficiency of our defences and, while we may relieve the toxic load by cleansing diets and stimulate our reserves with bathing or supplements, we need more specific side-effect free help for particular symptoms. Herbal and homoeopathic medicines can provide this safe and soothing support.

Some of the substances used both herbally and homoeopathically for hay fever are the same but their mode of action seems to be at different levels. Herbal medicines are prepared exclusively from plants — often from those whose pollens are such a problem to the hay fever victim — and their action is mainly a pharmacological one; that is the properties of the various substances in the herb bring about a chemical change in the body. Homoeopathic medicines on the other hand are prepared both from plant and mineral substances by a special process of dilution, known as potentization, and the final medicine will often contain no detectable trace of the original ingredient. The therapeutic benefit is achieved at a more subtle and, as yet, unexplained level.

The major advantage of herbal and homoeopathic medicines is their safety. If they are used in the appropriate way they are free from the side-effects so often associated with drugs, such as the antihistamines and aspirins. Natural medicines act by promoting the resistance, improving the drainage of the lymphatic system or sinuses, adjusting the functions of the lungs, and toning the mucous membranes. In many cases the medicinal action of the plant is safer because of the natural balance which is inherent in its composition, whereas the extraction of a purified active principle, which is sometimes done to produce drugs from plants, increases the likelihood of toxic effects because of the lack of vital buffering substances.

HERBAL MEDICINES

Herbal medicines are an ancient way of alleviating mankind's ailments which have stood the test of time through many centuries. With modern scientific techniques the long-recognized healing properties of herbs can be explained more accurately by their effects on the physiology.

One of the most valuable medicinal herbs is the Purple cone flower (Echinacea) which grows wild in the prairies of the U.S.A. and has long been cultivated in Europe for its medicinal properties. Scientific investigations have shown that it possesses mild antibiotic properties and specific immune-system stimulating effects, enhancing the function of the T-lymphocytes.

Preparing herbs

The most convenient way of taking herbs medicinally is as an infusion which may be prepared from the fresh plant or the dried herb. If you have access to the fresh plant, either in your own garden or by the wayside, then this is probably the best form in which to use it, but dried herbs may be purchased from herbal suppliers and some health food stores.

Use a pestle and mortar to gently crush the fresh plant or grind the dried herb to the consistency of tea or tobacco. You will need 30g of the dried herb or 80g of the fresh herb to 500ml of water. Pour boiling water over the herbs then cover the vessel and keep it in a warm place to steep for ten or fifteen minutes, stirring occasionally. Then strain and use the liquid in teacupful doses two or three times daily.

Another method is to use one teaspoonful of the dried herb in a cup of hot water.

Medicinal herbs for hay fever

Cone flower
(Echinacea angustifolia)

is invaluable for its tonic properties. It promotes the natural immunity, increases the general resistance, and is a blood purifier. Echinacea should be taken regularly from March or April onwards to build up resistance prior to the pollen season. It is frequently combined with other herbal medicines in the treatment of hay fever and general allergic disorders.

Coltsfoot
(Tussilago farfara)

is soothing and encourages the removal of phlegm which has obstructed the throat or chest. It helps to relax the spasm of the bronchi which causes wheezes.

Elderflower
(Sambucus nigra)

is diuretic and diaphoretic (promotes urination and sweating) and is, therefore, a valuable adjunct to cleansing programmes. It is often used in formulae for colds and catarrh and is useful for the hay fever case with a background of sinus congestion.

Eyebright
(Euphrasia officinalis)

is an essential herb for hay fever. When taken internally it soothes the irritable and inflamed throat or nose and especially the eyes. Drink the infusion three to four times daily. You may also cool the infusion to use for small compresses which may be placed over the eyelids while resting.

Garlic
(Allium sativum)

This is one of the outstanding herbal remedies for chronic catarrhal conditions. It is a natural antiseptic and blood purifier and combines well with Echinacea and Mullein for cleansing and detoxifying. The bulb is the most effective part of the plant but, apart from eating raw garlic in salads (if you don't have to socialize for at least 24 hours), garlic-oil capsules are available from health food stores. It is, however, best to take it in the form of dried garlic made up as tablets.

Golden Rod
(Solidago virgaurea)

is a stimulating slightly astringent tonic to the mucous membranes so it is particularly helpful in cases of catarrh with sneezing and excessive mucus.

Golden Seal
(*Hydrastis canadensis*)

is described by old herbalists as the king of tonics to the mucous membrane. It is restorative to irritated and inflamed membranes.

Hyssop
(*Hyssopus officinalis*)

is a classic cough medicine. It is also soothing to the inflamed membranes of the hay fever sufferer. (It should not be taken during pregnancy.)

Ma huang
(*Ephedra sinica*)

is a Chinese herb with antispasmodic properties of value to hay fever and asthma. Combine it with Echinacea (Cone flower) but use half the quantity (15g of the dried herb). Caution in high blood pressure, heart disease, and if on tranquillizers.

Mullein
(*Verbascum thapsus*)

soothes the bronchial tubes and mucous surfaces with slight astringent action to reduce excessive catarrh.

Pokeroot
(*Phytolacca decandra*)

is another valuable long-term remedy. Use it with Echinacea as a blood purifier. Poke root is particularly beneficial in cases of chronic congestion of the lymphatic tissues. Children with a tendency to swollen glands are often susceptible to allergies and Poke root, combined with other herbs, will gradually get them working more efficiently.

Red sage
(*Salvia officinalis*)

may be used as a mouth lotion or gargle for pharyngitis and sore throat. It is soothing and mildly antiseptic so it is of value for the treatment of mouth ulcers as well. May be combined with Myrrh (*Commiphora molmol*) for pharyngeal irritation.

Yarrow
(*Achillea millefolium*)

is a tonic to the membranes and induces perspiration. Especially useful with the onset of feverish symptoms.

Herbal compounds

You may combine several different herbs in an infusion to work on various aspects of your hay fever. The following combinations are often used according to the indications given:

- *To raise general resistance and tone the mucous membranes*
Cone flower, Pokeroot and Mullein
(start in early spring and continue throughout the hay fever season).

- *For general detoxification and cleansing diet adjunct*
Cone flower, Pokeroot, Elderflower, Mullein, and Yarrow.

- *For acute hay fever with itchy eyes and runny nose*
Cone flower, Euphrasia and Golden rod.

- *Tight chest, wheezy cough, with tenacious mucus*
Elderflower, Mullein, Hyssop, Yarrow, Coltsfoot, and Ma huang.

There are a number of commercially made preparations that are available from health food stores which are formulated from herbs together with vitamins. Others are prescribed by natural therapy practitioners, such as medical herbalists or naturopaths. The *Sambucus complex*, made by Blackmore Botanicals, contains Elderflower, Eyebright, Cone flower, and Golden Seal, with vitamins A and E, and is prescribed for rhinitis, hay fever, and other respiratory complaints with good effect. You should consult a naturopath or medical herbalist for more precise prescription of your individual needs.

HOMOEOPATHIC MEDICINES

Homoeopathy is based on the principle of 'like cures like'. The ideal medicine is an infinitesimal dose of the substance which would, in material quantity, cause the symptoms you wish to treat. Thus *Arsenicum*, a classic remedy of value for hay fever symptoms, is a preparation of a minute quantity of Arsenic trioxide which is a poison that would give severe burning and prickly symptoms in the membranes.

Homoeopathic medicines can be prepared from anything which causes the symptoms, and the most obvious choice would be to use the offending pollens, or other antigens. This has been done with some success, but the most commonly used homoeopathic medicines are made from medicinal plants and minerals which have a more general effect on body function. One part of the tincture of the medicinal substance is mixed with nine parts of distilled water and then shaken vigorously in a process known as potentization. This forms the first decimal potency, or 1x potency (shown in Europe and some other countries as 1D). This solution is then diluted one in ten to form the second decimal potency 2x, and so on. In centesimal potencies the dilution is one part to 99 parts, signified as 1c, 6c, and so on, but commonly with just the number after the name of the remedy, such as *Arsenicum* 6. The higher the potency the greater the power of the homoeopathic remedy.

For self-prescribing the 6th or 12th centesimal potencies are the best to work with. Homoeopathic remedies are available as tablets, or granules from homoeopathic pharmacies and some health food stores.

Homoeopathic research

Critics of homoeopathy are inclined to suggest that such infinitesimal quantities of the remedy cannot have any therapeutic power and that any benefit felt by patients is the result of the placebo effect (improvement due to belief rather than any active medicine). A research project to show that this is not so was reported in *The Lancet* of 18 October 1986 by Dr David Taylor Reilly and colleagues of the Glasgow Homoeopathic Hospital.

They compared the effects of a homoeopathic potency of mixed grass pollens (a preparation of the pollens of twelve species of grass potentized to 30c) with placebo tablets (dummy tablets with no medical ingredient).

The homoeopathically treated patients showed a significant improvement of their symptoms compared with those treated by the placebo. The homoeopathic group also used far less anti-histamines in the period of the trial which included peak pollen counts of over 300 grains per cubic millimetre.

Hay fever remedies

The selection of appropriate remedies for each individual is a matter for careful assessment by a qualified practitioner, but there are a number of well-tried remedies which, in the lower potencies, are perfectly safe to take and have been found to give relief to the acute symptoms of hay fever. Each remedy is known by the Latin name of its substance of origin, followed by the number which signifies the potency.

For a basic dose take one tablet three times daily. In acute situations a dose may be taken up to every half hour for four to five doses. Generally the frequency of dosage is reduced as symptoms improve. If there is any aggravation of symptoms on the basic dose, wait until improvement before repeating the dose. The aggravation may be a normal response to the remedy as it exerts its therapeutic power.

Do not bring any strong aromatic substances within close proximity of the remedy and do not take any food, drink, or use toothpaste within one hour of the dose as they may neutralize the medicinal effect.

Choose the most appropriate remedy according to the individual symptoms and your specific characteristics, such as preferences for warm or cold drinks, and whether or not the nasal discharge irritates. You may need different remedies at different stages of the season.

Allium cepa 6.   Streaming eyes and nose. Throat feels as if it tears on coughing. Nasal discharge is acrid but that from the eyes is bland.

Arsenicum album 12.   Burning or itchy eyes, inflamed nose and throat, streaming watery mucus. Good when acute symptoms have become established. A few half-hourly doses may give quick relief.

Euphrasia officinalis 6.   Itchy, sore eyes, but may be bland nasal discharge.

Natrum muriaticum 6.   Sinusitis and sneezes. A remedy for intermittent symptoms. It removes some of the susceptibility to sneezes and nasal congestion.

Pulsatilla 6.   Thicker nasal and sinus congestion with old green or yellow mucus, but bland. Gentle, tearful type of person without thirst but relieved by cold drinks.

Sabadilla 6.   Sneezes in open air, especially if cold. Sore nose, with tendency to bleed. Relieved by warm air. Symptoms aggravated by the odour of flowers.

Sinapis nigra 6.   Acrid discharge, nostrils tend to block alternately. Cough relieved by lying down.

Wyethia 12.   Indicated for the early symptoms of hay fever with sore itchy palate and pharynx and tickling at the back of the nose.

Homoeopathic combinations

Combinations of several homoeopathic remedies in one formula are commonly used. Many remedies are compatible in low potencies and the different facets of the problem are tackled simultaneously.

Many naturopaths, herbalists, and homoeopaths, use the Oligoplex (small dose complex) formulae from the famous Dr Madaus Herbal Institute of Germany. The *Sinapis nigra Oligoplex* contains Sinapis nigra 3x, Ailanthus 3x, Aralia 3x, Sabadilla 4x, Salix 2x, and Cepa 4x, and, when used with *Echinacea Oligoplex* containing Echinacea together with several other homoeopathic remedies, has given good relief to many thousands of hay fever sufferers. The Oligoplex preparations need prescribing by a practitioner familiar with the criteria for selecting the right remedy, but your health food store or a homoeopathic pharmacy may have other low-potency combinations helpful to hay fever sufferers.

BIOCHEMIC TISSUE SALTS

The Biochemic system of medicine was originated by Dr W.H. Scheussler, who recognized that the main solutions to disease lay within the body itself. The twelve Biochemic remedies, or Scheussler Tissue Salts, correspond to the principal inorganic elements found in the body, and he developed a system of prescribing based on homoeopathic principles.

The system differs from homoeopathy in that Scheussler devised it as a means of correcting disturbances of mineral salt metabolism. The distinction lies in the level at which the different types of medicine operate. Just as the herb Pokeroot is indicated for the same symptoms as its homoeopathic form, *Phytolacca*, so do the homoeopathic and biochemic forms of, for example, *Natrum muriaticum* have similar indications, but they all work in a slightly different way.

Of the twelve tissue salts there are four which have proved their worth in the management of hay fever. Biochemic tissue salts are generally potentized to 6x and all are available from health food stores as tablets.

which can be placed on or under the tongue to dissolve straight into the blood stream.

Take 4 tablets (children 2) 3-4 times a day for 1-2 months before the hay fever season and throughout the peak pollen times. For acute attacks 4 tablets every half hour will bring relief. Reduce the frequency of the doses as you improve.

Ferrum phos.   is indicated for inflamed burning sensations with congestion and headaches.

Natrum mur.   is for copious thin watery discharges, sneezing, and watery eyes. It can be alternated with Ferrum phos. Dr J.B. Chapman, in the book *Dr Scheussler's Biochemistry* (New Era Laboratories, 1961) recommends dissolving 15-20 tablets of Natrum mur. in warm water to use as a nasal wash.

Kali mur.   is helpful where the catarrh has become more thickened and where there are glandular swellings. May be alternated with Ferrum phos.

Kali phos.   relieves the asthmatic type of reaction to pollens with spasmodic cough. Helps to overcome the fatigue induced by the allergy and nourishes the nervous system.

Actions of the tissue salts

The chlorides, such as Kali mur. and Natrum mur. are stimulating and help to oxygenate tissues. Sodium (Natrum) is a distributing salt and helps to move excess fluid. Potassium (Kalium) salts are relaxing and relieve congestion.

Biochemic combinations

Many health food stores carry combinations of several biochemic tissue salts formulated for specific conditions. The New Era *Combination H* is composed of Magnesium phosphate 6x, Natrum mur. 6x, and Silica 6x, and gives safe and effective relief to many cases of hay fever and allergic rhinitis. Dosage is 4 tablets (children 2 tablets) 3 times a day or half hourly if required.

8 *Folk Remedies and Wonder Cures*

More than a grain of truth

Hay fever, like many other disorders, has its share of folklore remedies; simple measures which are said to have brought quick relief or cure. Such stories may have arisen from occasional spontaneous fluke responses of the body's defence system, or traditional measures found effective on a more consistent basis. Then there are the 'wonder cures', hailed in the health food trade as miracle nutrients with wide-ranging powers. Whether these claims are entirely justified is debateable, but it must be remembered that the remedies in question wouldn't have gained their reputations without some success to substantiate them.

The grain of truth common to them all may be that they each possess some ingredient, or combination of ingredients, that meets the individual needs of those who find them beneficial. Most of them have the ability to raise the general level of health and vitality; and this alone, in people who were hitherto very debilitated, would bring about a seemingly miraculous change. The difference may not be so striking in the healthy, well nourished person. The hay fever sufferer usually falls in the latter category; it is a complaint that can strike the otherwise apparently healthy individual. The fact that it does, however, indicates that there is some inadequacy in their body defence which might just be met by one of the constituents of the remedies described here.

Quite how helpful these foods or supplements are for hay fever is impossible to say, since most of them are still the subject of continuing research, and the benefits must be largely based on anecdote.

The industrious bee

The most promising group of remedies owe their potential for helping hay fever victims to the industriousness of the bee. These are the honey and pollen-related products. Bees spend a great deal of time among the pollens and they digest and distil out many vital substances which may be protective to our bodies. Apart from their inherent nutritional value, the 'potentization' of the pollens by the bees may impart benefit to the consumer of their products and stimulate, in particular, the defences against the effects of inhaled pollens.

Royal jelly

This glandular secretion of worker bees is so named because they feed it to female bee larvae destined to become queens. The workers are themselves female but have only fed on honey and pollen. The royal jelly is a much richer more concentrated nutrient with a high content of vitamins of the B complex, folic acid, and vitamin C, and is esteemed for its immune-enhancing properties. In its marketed form it is frequently combined with other nutrients and tonic foods, such as ginseng and vitamin E.

Honeycomb

Many people have reported that by consuming a small amount of pure honeycomb each day they have been able to keep hay fever at bay. A teaspoonful should be chewed each morning. Apart from providing immediate energy, as sucrose, comb honey will contain traces of pollen and other nutrients which may stimulate defence mechanisms.

Propolis

This is a sticky resin-like substance which bees collect from the coating of leaf buds on trees for lining and repairing their hives. Like royal jelly, some finds its way into the honey and through this its healing properties were discovered.

Propolis appears to possess natural antibiotic properties and has been found, by Professor Osmanagic of the University of Sarajevo in Yugoslavia, to be preventative against colds and influenza. It is highly likely to be of benefit in many cases of hay fever.

Pollen

Pollen extract is the ingredient of many tonic preparations available from health food stores. You might think that if you suffer from pollinosis the last thing you want to take is pollen, but there is a difference between swallowing it, to digest its natural nutrients, and inhaling it so that it penetrates sensitive nasal membranes. When it is used as a food supplement pollen is broken down to its basic nutrient composition which does not trigger the allergic response, if the digestive processes are working adequately.

Pollens vary in their nutritional content, but most contain important amino acids, vitamins A, D, E, and B-complex, and the minerals sodium, potassium, magnesium, calcium, zinc, and manganese. Pollen probably imparts valuable protective properties to the allergic individual and may be worthy of trial. It is available as dried pollen extract or capsules and is often incorporated with other tonics in special combinations.

Ginseng

Ginseng root has gained considerable fame as a tonic in recent years. It has long been a valued stimulant in traditional Chinese medicine where *Panax ginseng* was the species most commonly used, but the research which confirmed its health benefits has been conducted mostly in Russia, where Siberian ginseng (*Eleutherococcus senticosus*) originated. Ginseng, too, contains adaptogens which reintegrate body functions and stimulate the regenerative processes.

Ginseng is often incorporated in other tonic preparations, but it is also available in many other forms such as teas, granules, tablets, or the dried root. Pure Panax ginseng root is probably the most valuable form in which to take it. It is also the most expensive way to take it, but luckily you need only chew a thin slice each day.

Apple cider vinegar

This is prepared from apple cider and is not to be confused with malt vinegar which is more acidic. Cider is made by yeast fermentation of apple juice, then, after maturing, is allowed to undergo further fermentation by the action of *Acetobacter* which converts it to acetic acid. The cider vinegar is then diluted to bring the acetic acid content to 48 per cent before bottling. Some brands are preserved with vitamin C and others with sulphur dioxide.

Cider vinegar entered the 'wonder-food' league when D. C. Jarvis extolled its virtues for the treatment of rheumatic disorders in his book *Arthritis and Folk Medicine* (Pan, 1971) but it has all round value. Its properties seem to derive from a rich content of vitamins and minerals but, since many foods are equally good sources of these nutrients, there may be other factors to do with the acidic nature of the product which help us to use it advantageously. A dessertspoonful in warm water before meals can be beneficial to the digestion.

In *Hanssen's Complete Cider Vinegar* (Thorsons, 1974) Maurice Hanssen reports the case of a woman who was able to overcome her hay fever after suffering for thirty years, by taking two teaspoonsful of honey and cider vinegar in water every day throughout the season.

Evening primrose oil

The Evening primrose is a yellow-flowering plant whose seeds have been found to yield an oil with remarkable properties. These derive mainly from its content of the essential fatty acid, gammalinolenic acid (GLA). GLA comprises over ten per cent of the total essential fatty acid content of the Evening primrose.

Atopic or allergic individuals have been found to be deficient in an enzyme, Delta 6-desaturase, which converts the EFA linoleic acid to GLA on the way to forming the anti-inflammatory prostaglandin, PGE_1. With this enzyme deficiency there is a gradual decline in the production of PGE_1. The GLA already present in Evening primrose oil, however, bypasses this stage and, with the help of vitamins B, C, and minerals zinc, and magnesium, can produce the protective prostaglandin.

PGE_1 stimulates the T-lymphocytes, especially the T-suppressor cells which protect against exaggerated immune responses in hay fever.

Evening Primrose oil capsules are available from health food stores and should be taken at the maximum recommended dose throughout the hay fever season, although it would be beneficial to start at a lower dose early in the spring.

Molasses

Blackstrap molasses has been the subject of many health claims when used either as a drink (one teaspoonful in a cup of hot water) or as a sweetener on fruit salads or with muesli. Molasses, a product of an early stage in the refinement of sugar, is rich in minerals and trace elements, especially calcium and potassium. It is mildly laxative and something of a general tonic but not advisable as a regular food supplement for people with a tendency to low blood sugar.

Brewer's yeast

Brewer's yeast is rich in vitamins of the B complex and it contains up to twenty per cent of protein. It may usefully be taken as a supplemental food item to raise the general resistance of the hay fever sufferer and is valuable in the management of the low blood sugar syndrome.

Brewer's yeast is available from health food stores, either in tablet form or as the crude yeast which may be added to food. Don't confuse it with baking yeast.

Sea salt

Sodium plays an important part in the fluid balance of our bodies, and the benefits of homoeopathic and biochemic Natrum mur. (Sodium chloride) for hay fever have already been described. Pure sodium chloride, as found in normal table salt, is too concentrated for the body and leads to the retention of fluids as well as aggravating catarrhal states. Sea salt, because it contains other minerals and trace elements in a balanced form, is more acceptable and should be used in preference to table salt.

Sea salt may have preventative properties against hay fever. In the correspondence column of *The Guardian* on 16 June 1987, a reader, Mr Michael B. Rooke, of Durham, described how his hay fever subsided for 10-15 minutes after using sea salt with a meal. He found that by using a third of a teaspoonful on his breakfast cereal he was able to get almost a day's protection.

Spirulina

The ancient Aztecs of Mexico valued Spirulina for it's nutritional properties. Spirulina is a blue-green algae which grows on the surface of alkaline lakes and synthesizes food materials from the water and air using the energy of the sun.

Scientific research has shown that Spirulina is the richest natural source of protein yet discovered, with a content of over 65 per cent, compared with meat and fish at 18-20 per cent, cheese at 26 per cent, and Brewer's yeast at 20 per cent. It also contains other important nutrients, including vitamin B_{12}, vitamin A (equivalent to fish liver oil), and the vital prostaglandin precursor, gammalinolenic acid (GLA). Its GLA content matches that of Evening primrose oil.

Spirulina is filtered from the waters of Lake Taxacoco in Mexico, and is carefully dried before being formed into the tablets or powder which are available from your health food store. The powder may be used with fruit juices in the cleansing programmes as a valuable supplement for hay fever cases with low blood sugar tendencies.

Tonic combinations

There are a number of general tonics consisting of combinations of ingredients renowned for their health giving properties. Several manufacturers have combined Royal jelly with pollen, ginseng, and vitamin E. The quantities of each ingredient vary and you must be guided by the health food store proprietor.

The strongest tend to be the most expensive but they are the most effective. Royal jelly and Propolis are high quality products which are difficult to obtain so it is worth paying the price for a good brand. Propolis pastilles with eucalyptus may relieve the sore pharynx and nasal congestion associated with hay fever.

Which of the wonder cures for hay fever?

Without definitive research it is impossible to say which of these tonics will be especially helpful to hay fever sufferers. Some are likely to be of direct benefit and are definitely worthy of trial, and others, while having general health giving properties, may be regarded as 'optional extras' to use from time to time. The following table may be of some guidance.

Definitely worth a try	Optional extras
Pollen extract	Propolis
Royal jelly	Apple cider vinegar
Honeycomb	Brewer's yeast
Sea salt	Molasses
Ginseng	
Evening primrose oil	
Spirulina	

9 *Nature's Gifts*

Water, air, and sunlight

Water, air, and natural daylight are essential to us all; they are life's necessities and we can also regard them as nature's gifts. All living things depend on them, including the plants that plague you with their pollens, but they may also be used to promote healing. It is an example of making nature work for you rather than fighting it.

Water is versatile and vital to life. It can transform from liquid to solid ice or vapour, and acts as a carrier of many essential substances in all three forms. Its capacity to transmit or absorb heat is one of its most valuable properties for the hay fever sufferer. This is the basis of its use in hydrotherapy, where baths, packs, and compresses are applied to stimulate the circulation.

Mineral waters, from various spas, contain essential elements in an ionic form which are more readily absorbed either through the skin or in the digestive system when they are swallowed. These minerals may act as catalysts to biochemical processes in the body.

Air is also an important stimulant of vitality. It is, of course, the provider of essential oxygen, and full free breathing is important to good health and body defence. We shall consider this more fully in Chapter 11.

Sunlight, or natural daylight, is also known to play a vital role in promoting the immunity of the body, apart from being necessary to our assimilation of vitamin D.

Skin — the vital organ

Nearly all the benefits nature's gifts confer on us happen through the medium of the skin. The skin has blood vessels and nerve endings which react to the stimuli of water, air, and sunlight, and through reflex connections, influence the function of internal organs, such as the lungs. According to traditional Chinese medicine the skin is closely related to the lungs and the whole respiratory system so it is not simply because of an allergic disposition that problems such as hay fever, asthma, and eczema, often go together.

As far as hay fever is concerned the most significant function of the skin is as an eliminative organ. Perspiration is similar in composition to urine. Up to one third of the body's waste matter may be eliminated through the skin and we may sweat off as much as a pound of impurities in a day. The skin clearly needs to be made to work with more efficiency, and yet we cosset and cover our bodies so that they are given little opportunity to breathe and eliminate adequately.

Some people also spend a fortune on deodorants and anti-perspirants which anaesthetize the pores. The journey to work on the tube and bus might be a lot less agreeable were it not for these, but the price of health does not necessarily have to be the loss of one's friends and neighbours. The introduction of tonic measures for the skin and the adoption of a diet containing less refined foods will reduce the problems of body odour in many cases.

There are many tonic measures which help to promote better skin function, such as dry brushing, friction rubs, sprays, and compresses. Even exposing the skin to the cool air from time to time has a tonic effect.

The skin is also capable of absorbing mineral and medicinal substances. Essential oils and homoeopathic medicines in solution may be rubbed on to the skin on the inside of the wrist or forearm and will be taken up by the blood in the fine vessels beneath the surface.

One of the simplest and finest stimulants of skin function is dry skin brushing.

Dry skin brushing

This is a most beneficial and pleasant way of toning skin function. The friction of the bristles rubs off dead cells on the body surface and clears the pores as well as stimulating the circulation. You will need a natural bristle brush; nylon is too harsh. Some pharmacies and hardwear stores have bath brushes of natural bristle with detachable handles that enable you to reach the middle of your back.

Start with the hands or feet and work up the limbs towards the trunk with a brisk to-and-fro or circular action. Then move onto the trunk, avoiding only the face and areas of sensitive or inflamed skin. Continue until you feel a warm glow all over the body. Shower or rinse down with cool or tepid water and dry with a rough towel.

HYDROTHERAPY

There are many ways of using water to promote well-being ranging from its application to the skin as packs, compresses, baths, and sprays, to the taking of mineral-rich spa waters, and the colon cleansing procedures, such as enemas.

Most of the applications described here will be of assistance to the hay fever sufferer in some way and all are capable of being done in your own home with very little equipment.

Water sniffing

This simple procedure can give some relief to the prickly, inflamed nasal passages. Immerse the nostrils in cold water scooped in the palms of your hands, sniff it up and allow it to run out again. Don't worry if some goes back into the pharynx at the back of the mouth. It can be swallowed or spat out.

The cold water cools and constricts the vessels in the congested membranes. This should be used as an emergency relief measure only which you may do several times a day but it is best not repeated too frequently or you may remove natural protective mucous.

Saline irrigation

Some medical trials report significant improvement in the symptoms of allergic rhinitis following treatment with a special preparation of physiological saline. Other reports of the benefits of sea salt on hay fever symptoms (see page 101) suggest that the addition of small amounts of sea salt to water used for bathing the nasal membranes may be of value.

Steam inhalation

For the stuffy congested nose, and especially where catarrh is difficult to shift, steam inhalation is beneficial. Warm moist air counteracts the effects of cold air on sensitive noses. An experiment reported in the *American Review of Respiratory Disease* (No. 135, June 1986) showed that patients with allergic rhinitis who inhaled cold dry air produced significantly greater amounts of the leukotrienes (chemical mediators of allergy similar to histamine in their effects on the membranes) than when they inhaled warm moist air. Various other medical reports have confirmed the benefits of warm vapour in the relief of nasal sensitivity.

Place a bowl containing boiling water on a table then sit with your head over the bowl covered with a large towel. Breathe in and out deeply, inhaling the steam. The vapour loosens mucus in the respiratory tract, an effect that will be enhanced by adding a few drops of *Olbas*, or other aromatic oils to the water.

Special inhalation equipment is available from some chemists and medical supply shops.

The wet friction rub

This is another method, similar to the dry brushing, of promoting the eliminative functions of the skin. It is a slightly stronger stimulus because of the use of cold water with the friction. It speeds up removal of dead cells on the surface, clears the pores, and promotes the circulation.

After a bath or shower rub down the whole body with a loofah, or a string or friction glove available from a chemist, soaked in cold water. Start with the extremities, working upwards towards the trunk then rub down the trunk using brisk to-and-fro movements. Try to achieve a pleasant glow on the skin.

Friction rubs should not be done over areas of eczema or other rashes or where the skin is broken.

The *salt rub* is another method of skin friction which can be done in a shower. Soak the body with warm or cold water then, using large containers of salt, rub down the whole skin surface, except the face, using the wet salt in your hands for the friction.

Enemas

The most suitable enema for home use is the gravity feed type which can be obtained from any reputable chemist. It consists of a canister which holds two or three pints of water, and a long rubber tube leading from the base of this to a plastic tap device. A nozzle, known as a catheter, is supplied and this should be attached to the tap.

The canister should be filled with water which has been warmed to just above body temperature (to about 100°F/38°C). For children you will require half to one pint, according to age, and for adults two pints of water. Hang the canister at a reasonable height, for example on the back of the bathroom door. The catheter should be lubricated with some vaseline or olive oil smeared around the end but keeping the aperture clear.

The enema is best administered in the knee-chest position, that is kneeling down and resting forwards on the elbows, but if you are giving it to yourself it would be more convenient to lie on your back or on the left side. Insert the catheter gently to its full length (less with children). Turn the tap on to allow the water to flow in. If there is any discomfort while the water is flowing into the rectum it may be due to pressure of pockets of wind. Stop the flow by turning off the tap or pinching the rubber tube, knead the abdomen with the hand until the pain has dispersed and then allow the water to continue to flow in. When all the water has flowed in or you have taken all that you can hold, withdraw the catheter gently.

Before evacuating, lie on your back with knees bent for five minutes and gently knead the abdomen to allow the water to move about and soften any hardened faecal matter.

Enemas should not be administered when on a full diet nor should they be taken too frequently. A small enema once daily during an acute febrile illness is permissible but they should only be necessary on isolated occasions at other times.

Contrast bathing

Bathing areas of the body with water of contrasting temperatures promotes better circulation to the areas treated. The warm application dilates the blood vessels and relaxes the pores and other surface tissues. The cold application, which immediately follows it, then causes the contraction of the small vessels, and, as blood drains away from the area, the local congestion is relieved. The rate of removal of waste products is increased and fresh blood brings more oxygen to the area.

Hot and cold splashes

This is an effective treatment for nasal congestion and stuffiness. It relieves a headache due to catarrh of the sinuses.

Splash or sponge the whole face with warm water for one to two minutes then with cold water for half to one minute. Repeat four to five times finishing with the cold application.

Hot and cold foot baths

These balance the circulation of the whole body and relieve congestion of the head and sinuses.

Use two bowls and fill one with hot water and the other with cold. Place the feet in the bowl of hot water and soak for three minutes then plunge them in the cold water keeping them there for one minute. Repeat this process for ten to fifteen minutes finishing with the cold application.

As an alternative you may spray or sponge the legs and feet with hot and cold water. Spraying the lower legs and feet with cold water only for two or three minutes before retiring is conducive to good sleep.

Baths

Warm baths relax the vessels of the skin surface and open the pores while contrast baths of the whole or part of the body can also be beneficial. It can also be a good way of delivering various herbal and mineral substances to the blood via the skin.

Epsom salts baths

The Epsom salts bath is a valuable eliminative treatment. It draws heat to the surface of the body, dilates the pores, and increases perspiration. It is a useful adjunct to the cleansing programme.

Place a heaped double handful of commercial Epsom salts in a bath of hot water (99-108°F/37-42°C). Use the purified Epsom salts available in cheaper and larger quantities from some chemists or garden centres. Soak in the bath, immersed up to the neck, for fifteen to twenty minutes. Place a cold compress on the forehead.

Get out slowly in case of light headedness, rinse down with cool or tepid water and dry with a rough towel. If you can get straight into bed wrap a bath towel or sheet around you and allow the perspiration to continue. Later you may rub down with a cold wet flannel, or sponge, and dry with a warm rough towel.

Herbal baths

Various herbal substances can be used in therapeutic baths. Hayflowers are a selection of meadow grasses and wild flowers, from which an infusion is made to add to the warm bath. Oat straw baths were recommended by Father Sebastian Kneipp, the nineteenth century German pioneer of hydrotherapy, for promoting the functions of the kidneys and bladder. Various aromatic oils such as pine oil and rosemary can be pleasant and soothing when added to the bath water.

Sitz baths

Sitz baths originated in the German spas where hydrotherapy is widely used. They act on the pelvic areas and abdomen being tonic to the intestines and, therefore, promoting bowel function. Drawing blood to the abdomen also helps to relieve the congestion of the head.

Proper sitz baths require specially designed hip baths but you can improvize with a large bowl or baby bath in your main bath tub. Place tolerably hot water in the bowl and cold water in the bath. The bowl of hot water can be placed in the bath. Sit in the hot water, with your feet in the cold water, for three minutes. Then change round to sit in the cold water, with your feet in the bowl of hot water, for one minute. Repeat three times. While sitting massage the hips and lower abdomen.

Packs and compresses

Throat compress

For sore or inflamed throats, swollen glands, loss of voice, or catarrh, the cold compress to the throat can bring quick relief. It promotes the circulation and increases the efficiency of the lymph glands and ducts in the area.

Wring out a man's handkerchief in cold water from the tap, squeeze well, then shake out surplus moisture. Fold lengthwise and place around the throat. Pin a woollen scarf round it to hold it in place.

The compress warms up within half an hour and can be kept on for two or three hours or overnight. It should be dry by the morning. If it remains cold or does not dry overnight it was probably not sufficiently squeezed out. The throat compress is best used with the trunk pack or abdominal pack.

Trunk pack

This is an excellent treatment for most feverish conditions and to promote the eliminative functions of the skin during cleansing programmes. The initial stimulus of the cold pack is followed by an increase of the circulation of the body surface with perspiration. This helps to relieve internal congestion, wherever it may be, and the temperature will be reduced. Use it with throat compresses for any fever and also as an aid to elimination in conjunction with the Fast Relief Plan, or other cleansing diet.

You will need a thin cotton sheet wide enough to wrap around the body at double thickness from the armpits to the groin; another sheet and a thick towel or blanket, both a little wider than the first. Babies' cot sheets are usually suitable and can be folded to size for smaller children.

Lay the towel or blanket on the bed with the spare sheet on top of it and the greater part of the spare length hanging over the side. Soak the other sheet in cold water, squeeze it out well and shake well, fold to the right width, then place it over the dry ones (a). Lie down on the wet sheet (b) then wrap the longer side around your trunk, rolling over if necessary to tuck it in and then fold the other side to overlap at the front or side of the body (c). Next wrap around the dry sheet and finally the blanket or towel, pinning the latter in place along the side with two or three safety pins (d). Slip pyjamas or nightdress over the pack and cover yourself with the bedclothes.

The pack should begin to warm up within fifteen minutes, but if it is still cool after half an hour it may have been put on too wet or the vital response may be insufficient to react and it should be taken off. When you take off a trunk pack, sponge down with cool or tepid water and then dry with a warm rough towel. You can check packs on children by putting your fingers between the pack and the body.

Normally the pack can be kept on for at least three hours and possibly overnight. It may induce perspiration, and where there is a good reaction it will dry out completely. Any dampness may only be due to perspiration

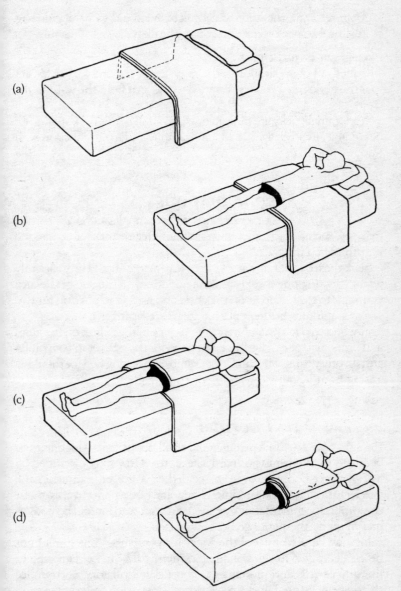

Figure 7. How to apply a trunk pack.

and, on removal, the inner sheet might be found to be discoloured by toxic substances secreted through the skin.

Abdominal or waist pack
The method of application is the same as for the trunk pack except that the abdominal pack is confined to the area from the waist to the groin.

Abdominal packs are indicated where a full trunk pack might not be suitable; in a younger child, for example, and in conjunction with throat compresses.

Fomentations

Fomentations are wet applications of thicker material, such as a towel. Hot fomentations relieve internal congestion in asthmatic attacks.

Soak the towel in hot water — from the hot tap should be sufficiently warm — wring out surplus moisture and fold to the size of the area you want to treat. Place it on the chest and leave it in position for two or three minutes before replacing it. Don't let it get too cool.

Hot and cold fomentations are more tonic in their effect on the lungs and bronchial tubes as well as being good for the relief of stiff or painful areas in other parts of the body; for example, an aching neck or shoulders arising from laboured breathing or coughing.

Thermal packs

These are liquid filled plastic bags which may be obtained from chemists or hardware stores. They can be warmed up in hot water or in an oven, or cooled in a freezer, and retain the temperature for a longer time. They are not as effective as moist compresses or fomentations as the beneficial reaction of the body is prevented by the prolonged cooling effect.

Ice may be used to cool the water for compresses but should not be applied direct to the skin. The extreme cold can be damaging to the surface cells and prevents the beneficial circulatory reaction. Ice should only be used under professional supervision for extreme cases of inflammation.

AIR

Cool air is a tonic stimulus to the skin, but there are few hay fever sufferers who can gain much pleasure from being in the fresh air during the summer.

Some of the benefits, traditionally attributed to fresh air in mountainous regions and beside the sea, may, in fact, be due to the higher concentration of negative ions in these regions. Negative ions are formed when molecules of oxygen, nitrogen, and carbon dioxide in the atmosphere gain electrons and become negatively charged. People with hay fever, and asthma, are greatly helped by negative ions. They reduce pollen levels in the atmosphere and histamine levels in the blood.

Machines which generate negative ions are available for home or office and these are described in Chapter 12.

SUNLIGHT

Natural light affects our health in several surprising ways. It is not only the radiant heat of sunlight which makes us feel better and helps us to produce vitamin D, but the full spectrum of normal daylight appears to have an essential role in stimulating body functions.

Light is the visible part of a spectrum of energy of differing wavelengths ranging from cosmic rays and x-rays at one end to radio and electric waves at the other. The visible portion is natural light which includes the spectrum of primary colours. Artificial light, especially that produced by fluorescent strip lights, consists of only the shorter wavelengths in a narrow part of the light spectrum, and many people who work for long periods under these have a higher incidence of health problems, including allergies.

In his book *Health and Light* (Pocket Books, New York, 1973) John N. Ott describes how full spectrum light may affect our health. He overcame his own arthritic problems by a programme of progressively longer exposure to natural light and recounts how a colleague did the same for his hay fever. Full spectrum light appears to work through the skin, and the eyes, affecting the pituitary gland, the 'master gland' which regulates many bodily functions.

You should try to ensure that you get plenty of exposure to natural daylight, even if the sun isn't shining. This may be more problematic when the pollens are around, so take advantage of the opportunity for being out at other times of the year. If you work under fluorescent lighting try to persuade your employer to install the full-spectrum fluorescent tubes which are available. These are closer to natural daylight than the shorter wavelength, cool-white lights. Full spectrum tubes cost a little more but they give better light and last longer. A noticeable reduction in allergies and other health problems has been reported when people working under full spectrum light are compared to those working in normal fluorescent light.

Colour

The individual colours within the light spectrum are believed to have an effect on health, knowledge of which may be used in choosing decor and as a form of treatment. This will be described in Chapter 13.

10 *Hands On for Hay Fever*

Massage and reflex treatments

Nobody realized quite how important touch is to man and animals until it was noticed that people with pets tend to live longer and have a lower incidence of disease. Then some famous psychological studies showed that baby monkeys, deprived of physical contact with their mothers, soon became ill and stunted in growth when compared to those who had the normal warmth and affection of a parent. There is no doubt that we all need the closeness, contact, and caring of fellow humans or animals.

Touch is comforting and calming and, when done with diligence, shows the concern of one creature for another, according to Doris Krieger Ph.D., RN, who, in 1972, was also able to show in a controlled trial that what she called Therapeutic Touch, resulted in an increase of haemoglobin, the oxygen-carrying pigment of the blood. This type of contact is natural for many health care professionals, especially nurses, but it finds its most beneficial expression in the various forms of massage and reflex therapy.

The hands are a powerful therapeutic tool used either by a trained therapist or even on yourself. There are many manual techniques which can help to alleviate the miseries of hay fever and improve general well-being and we shall look at some simple massage methods, reflex treatments to body and feet, and the use of medicinal oils, known as aromatherapy.

MASSAGE
Massage must be the oldest form of treatment known to man. Whenever we rub a tender spot we are giving a form of massage. It is a most pleasing experience to receive a massage and its benefits are far reaching. When applied appropriately it can give relief to hay fever as well as promoting the general metabolism.

The effects of massage are psychological, mechanical, physiological, and reflex.

Mechanical benefits. Its special benefits to the hay fever sufferer arise from its promotion of lymphatic drainage and circulation. The squeezing of muscles and tissues creates positive and negative pressures which stimulate the capillaries, yet stretches muscles and helps to improve the breathing. Massage also promotes skin perspiration and elimination by the friction and increase of blood flow.

The physiological effects of massage may also account for its *psychological* benefits and result from its reflex actions. There is an increased secretion of endorphins and enkephalins, hormones released by the brain which reduce pain and inflammation and bring about mood improvements.

The reflex effects arise from stimulation of nerve endings in the skin which then send impulses to the spinal cord from where messages pass out along other nerve pathways to the organs supplied by the same segment. This would appear to be the mechanism by which the various forms of reflex treatment, such as foot reflexology, and endocrine reflex therapy work. It may also account for the healing benefits of acupressure and shiatsu, although these are believed to work on a separate system of energy channels within the body which are the basis of the acupuncture system.

How to give massage
Massage is a specialized skill with many variations and refinements of technique to meet specific situations. You will benefit greatly from the services of a trained masseur, but it is possible for everyone to learn a few basic strokes to use on themselves, or their family and friends. It is a pleasant way of sharing, caring, and communicating.

There are several essentials to remember when giving a massage:

- The hands need to be warm.
- The hands should be relaxed but positive in their actions.
- Let the hands and fingers *mould* to the parts you are treating.

Use a little vegetable oil, such as sunflower seed or almond oil, or a special massage oil to lubricate the skin. Anoint the part you wish to treat with sufficient oil to prevent friction.

Massage is given with a variety of movements, the most useful of which are stroking, kneading, and stretching.

Stroking, or gliding, is done with the palms of the hands which are moved upwards on the limbs or trunk towards the heart in a steady rhythm. Exert a little more pressure on the upward glide, stroking lightly as you come downwards again. Use one hand, or both, on the arms and lower legs and both hands on the thighs and trunk or back.

This may be combined with *kneading* in which the fingers or heel of the hand are used to squeeze and stretch the skin and underlying flesh. Use thumb and fingers in a gentle pinch and roll manoeuvre on small areas, or fingers and heels of hands in bigger areas. When kneading try to move the skin over the underlying tissues moving on

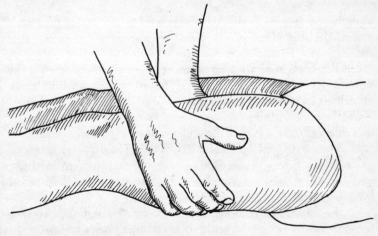

Figure 8. Allow the hands to mould comfortably to the parts you are treating.

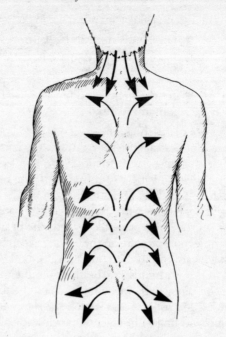

Figure 9. Direction for massage strokes on the back.

to each area as you do so. As you become used to using the hands you will be able to feel which strokes are appropriate in each part of the body.

On the back, start with broad moves away from the spine in an upwards and outwards direction, then follow on with smaller circular kneadings in tight or tender areas.

On the neck and shoulders you should work downwards in smaller movements from the base of the skull towards the shoulders and upper back. Massage of the neck, shoulders, and back is particularly helpful to hay fever sufferers because it promotes better circulation to the throat and sinuses, relaxes the muscles and improves the freedom of the breathing.

On the chest slow firm movements downwards and outwards to follow the lines of the ribs and muscles between them helps to release the breathing mechanisms and has reflex effects on major lymph vessels.

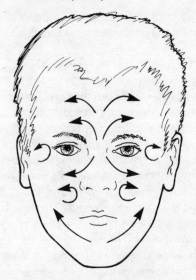

Figure 10.   Direction for massage strokes on the face.

The face can be massaged with smaller strokes using circular motions working out from the centre with thumbs or fingers. Start with the forehead and work upwards before moving to the nose, with strokes out to the cheekbones. This helps to relieve congestion of the nose and sinuses.

REFLEX TECHNIQUES

This electrical circuitry of our bodies — the nerves and energy pathways by which the messages are passed between one part and another — is complex, and we probably understand only a small part of its workings. What we do know is that impulses from the skin can travel, via the spinal cord, to other organs and zones of the body. These phenomena can be explained by the structure and distribution of the nerves.

There are also other remote effects which can be achieved by applying stimuli to more precise zones, or points, which may exert their influence by means of some energy system, such as the acupuncture channels, or by other, as yet undiscovered, nerve pathways. Whatever the scientific explanations for their effects you can make use of these reflex points to improve the functions concerned with breathing and the immune system.

Different reflex therapies have been developed by individuals in various cultures and it is probable that some of the oldest systems of medicine, such as acupuncture, developed from the application of these principles. George Chapman, an American osteopath, for example, discovered a number of areas of muscle fibre contraction, or trigger points, which are consistently associated with problems in organs and connected by nerve pathways via the spinal cord. Treating these areas of contraction, or ganglia, can improve the function of the glands and tissues, such as the tonsils and the sinuses. In China and Japan the twin systems of acupressure and shiatsu were evolved. They are both methods of treating special areas on the body surface, many of which correspond to major acupuncture points. The effect of pressure or massage to these points appears to be an adjustment of the body's self-regulating processes, possibly owing in part to the release of endorphins which they induce. Many points have a more direct influence on the nose and sinuses.

Hay fever reflex workout

All these systems have a lot of areas in common, so to avoid confusion I have selected a number of the most influential points to provide a Hay Fever Reflex Workout. Some of these reflex areas are acupoints, known by their Chinese names or a number, and others are named by the target organ with which they are connected. I have, therefore, given each one a new code number keyed roughly according to its anatomical location, which, with the help of the diagram, will make them easier to identify. The actions and locations of these special points are described in the table.

Select three or four points to work on at a session, using those which meet the immediate symptoms, as well as some to raise general resistance. For example, a suitable regular treatment might be the use of points F1, F2, F5, and L2. You may work on the main facial points several times a day and try to treat a selection of the body harmonizing points at least three times a week.

Use the tip of a finger or thumb applying pressure in a firm upward or circular kneading motion. Work according to the direction indicated for each point for half to one minute before moving on to the next

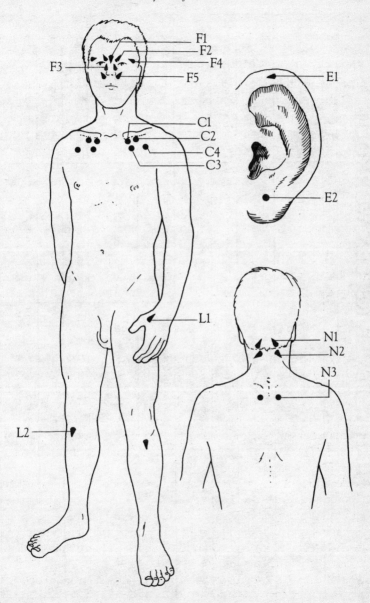

Figure 11. The hay fever reflex work out (see table for details).

THE HAY FEVER REFLEX WORKOUT

KEY	TYPE OF POINT	LOCATION	INDICATIONS	METHOD
F points are on the face				
F1	Acupuncture point *Yintang*	Above the bridge of the nose midway between the eyebrows in the position of the third eye.	Congestion and irritation of eyes, nose, and sinuses.	Massage with fingertip in downward direction.
F2	Acupoint	At the inner margin of the eyebrows on the bony ridge of the eye socket.	Congestion of sinuses, irritation and watering of eyes.	Pressure upwards and outwards with fingertips or thumbs.
F3	Acupoint	At the side of the bridge of the nose where the spectacles rest.	Nasal congestion and irritation.	Upwards in a circular motion.
F4	Acupoint *Tae yang*	Half inch behind the lateral margin of the eyebrow in the temporal depression.	Headache and sinus congestion.	Pressure forwards with fingertips.
F5	Acupoint	Just lateral to the fleshy part of the nostrils where they meet the crease formed when you smile.	Nasal congestion and irritation. Sinus congestion.	Circular massage upwards and outwards.
C points are on the chest				
C1	Chapman Reflex and acupoint	Beneath the inner end of the collar bone where it meets the sternum.	Nasal problems.	Circular kneading with thumb or fingertip.
C2	Chapman Reflex	Just lateral to C1.	Irritation and congestion of pharynx.	Circular kneading with fingertip.
C3	Chapman Reflex	Beneath C1 between the first and second ribs.	Tonsil congestion.	Circular kneading with thumb or fingertip.
C4	Chapman Reflex and acupoint	Three and a half inches from the sternum on the upper edge of the second rib.	Sinus irritation and congestion.	Circular kneading.

KEY	TYPE OF POINT	LOCATION	INDICATIONS	METHOD
N points are on the neck and back				
N1	Chapman and acupoint	Depression below the skull on the neck level with mastoid bone.	Headache, sinus congestion, and sore throat.	Circular kneading up and in.
N2	Chapman Reflex	Follow line of jaw round to back of neck on each side below N1.	Nasal irritation and congestion.	Circular kneading down and outwards.
N3	Acupoint	On the back one and a half inches from the midline just below the third thoracic spinous process. (Count four down from the most prominent at the top of the back with the neck bent.)	Lungs to tone and relieve spasm.	Firm circular kneading with thumbs.
Limbs				
L1	Acupoint	Back of the hand in the fleshy angle between thumb and first finger.	Clears head and nasal congestion.	Knead upwards with thumb. Use regularly.
L2	Acupoint	Just below knee in the angle at the top of the shin bone.	General tonic and boost to immunity.	Knead downwards. Use regularly.
Ear				
E1	Acupoint	Just below the tip of the ear on outer side of the overhang.	Allergy point.	Use corner of fingernail to massage forwards on the left and backwards on the right.
E2	Acupoint	Right in the centre of the fleshy lobe of the ear (often pierced for ear-rings).	Eye point for all weakness and irritation.	Corner of the nal. Place thumb behind the lobe and work against it.

pair. All points except those in the centre line have to be treated bilaterally.

Foot and hand reflexes

In 1935 Dwight C. Byers, who suffered annual bouts of asthma and hay fever, was visiting his aunt who was a therapist for a local physician in Conesus Lake, in upper New York State. She worked on his feet and soon he found relief for the first time ever.

Dwight's aunt was Eunice Ingham who became interested in the theories of Dr William Fitzgerald, the pioneer of reflex zone therapy. She developed her own ideas on foot reflexes and evolved them into the therapeutic system excellently described by Dwight Byers in his book *Better Health With Foot Reflexology* (Ingham Publishing Inc., St Petersburg, Florida, 1985).

The feet and hands have extensive reflex connections with the rest of the body. As might be expected of their importance in our evolution, they are richly supplied with nerve endings — the hands to provide us with the very tools which which we treat these reflexes, apart from the many other functions of which they are capable, and the feet as our means of contact with the earth's energy. But there are subtle nerve connections with every organ in the body and it is their representative zones on the soles and tops of the feet which give us a further means of influencing the function of areas such as the sinuses, lymph vessels, and intestines.

Although the whole body is represented on the soles of the feet and the palms of the hands, the areas shown in the chart are the main ones you will need to work on to promote the health of the respiratory organs and maintain general well-being. It would, nevertheless, be beneficial to obtain treatment from a trained and experienced foot reflexologist, who would detect the zones most in need of attention, including those which may indirectly affect your hay fever.

How to treat foot zones

You can work on your own feet at any convenient time with kneading movements of the fingertips or knuckles. Always work on the bare feet though you may apply pressure through socks if there isn't time to take them off. Grasp the foot from above and work on the zone with the tips of the fingers using squeezing and kneading motions. Work on each zone, or group of zones, for two to three minutes or until any tenderness or gritty feeling has diminished, then move on to the next area.

The balls of the feet may become quite fibrous and the crystalline deposits which you may feel will not disperse at one session so do not overdo the treatment and make the foot sore. If you are working on a friend's feet do not be tempted to do too much at a time, especially on tender areas. Over-stimulation of sensitive areas can be upsetting to the system in general.

Foot zones to treat for hay fever

Sinuses

On the pads of the four smaller toes are reflex zones for all sinus areas and membranes, so treat regularly to improve resistance or for congestion and irritation. Work with four fingers on the pads of the small toes simultaneously.

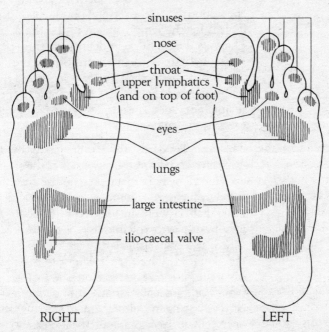

Figure 12. Foot reflex zones for hay fever.

Nose

Middle third of the ball of the great toe. Work in a circular motion for all nasal sensitivity and catarrh.

Throat

One third of the way up from the base of the great toe on the under surface. For the tonsils and pharyngeal region. Work from the inside to the outside of the toe with squeezing and stroking movements.

Lungs

Situated across the outer two thirds of the ball of the foot and on the upper surface above the roots of the toes. Use upward and circular kneading over the whole lung zone to improve the function of the bronchial tubes and relieve tendencies to coughs and wheezes.

Upper lymphatics

In the angle between the root of the great toe and the second toe on the top and bottom of the foot. This is for the lymph system of the throat and pharyngeal area. Efficient drainage of these ducts is essential to removal of impurities from the area. The tonsils are the first line of defence and they, with the whole lymph system, are important in maintaining adequate immunity. Knead upwards towards the ankle.

Colon

This zone lies across the middle just below the 'waistline' and down the outer side of the sole on each foot. The right foot represents the ascending colon and part of the transverse colon, and the other half is represented in the left foot. An important part of the intestines is the ileo-caecal valve between small and large intestine which must function freely for adequate elimination. Its zone lies at the lower end of the colon zone on the right foot. Work gradually around the colon zone on both feet giving special attention to any congestion or crystalline deposits around the ileo-caecal valve zone.

AROMATHERAPY

Among the preparations used by the ancient Egyptians for the mummification process, to preserve the bodies of their pharaohs, were oils which had antiseptic properties. The use of such essential oils therapeutically has been developed in the twentieth century as the science and art of aromatherapy.

Oils are prepared from the leaves, barks, roots, and seeds of various plants. Because large quantities of the raw material are needed to provide a small amount of oil it is an expensive preparation, but a little goes a long way. Essential oils can be used for massage or inhalation.

For massage you may add three or four drops of the appropriate oil to an eggcupful of vegetable oil, such as sunflower or almond oil. One or two drops of essential oil may be added to the hot water used for steam inhalation.

To find which oils would be most suitable for your specific needs you should consult a trained aromatherapist, but the following may be helpful for your hay fever on a first-aid basis.

Eucalyptus oil.	Suitable for inhalation to clear congested sinuses. Also massage into the facial areas especially the reflex points F1, F3, and F5 on the forehead and around the nose (see page 121).
Hyssop oil.	Antiseptic and expectorant which loosens chronic catarrh. Work it into the upper back and chest especially zones C1-C4 and N3.
Bergamot, Chamomile, and Lavender oils.	Stimulate the white blood cells and increase resistance. Chamomile contains a good anti-inflammatory ingredient, azulene. Use these oils especially on areas around the neck, back, and chest.

11 *Breathing Freely*

Exercise to tone the tubes

Our bodies were built for activity. They need it to maintain maximum function of skin, lungs, bowels, and kidneys. Exercise promotes the eliminative functions and stimulates the circulation. On the other hand we also need adequate sleep for cell replenishment and healing, but there is a difference between proper sleep and indolence.

There is nothing quite so conducive to poor vitality as inertia. It leads to a sluggishness of body functions which soon undermines resistance and makes us easy targets for infections and allergies. Without vigorous exercise we don't use our lungs to their maximum capacity. The deepest branches of the bronchioles, the fine tubes which terminate in the air sacs, are worked only very gently so the mucus they produce tends to accumulate and form a focus for infections. Even in the nose and sinuses the habit of breathing shallowly will leave some membranes under-oxygenated.

As a regular hay fever victim you may, by now, be wondering what sense there is in breathing more deeply if you are going to inhale a lot more pollens. Certainly, at the height of summer, that would be a problem. During the peak pollen months you may need to curb vigorous exercise in the open air and work indoors, in a gym, or at home, in a room with filters or ionizers. Alternatively, work out on wet days when the counts are low which may, at least, reduce the concentration of the pollens you inhale. You can also take advantage of the pollen-free times of year to build up your general fitness.

Exercise and well-being

The aim of the hay fever sufferer is not to attain peak athletic performance, but to be able to sustain optimum well-being. Exercise can make a positive contribution to this through promoting lung function and increasing elimination through the skin, as well as developing muscle flexibility, strength, and endurance.

A varied programme of aerobic exercise (in which muscles work to convert food to energy-using oxygen) is most suitable to meet these requirements. This develops heart and lung fitness in a gradual way. Walking and running are good aerobic exercises but swimming, or other indoor activity with rowing machines or exercise bicycles, may be more manageable when pollens abound.

Breathing effectively

Brisk exercise which makes you pant is the best way of getting air to all corners of the lungs and sinuses. This may not always be convenient so it is worth learning to breathe correctly for its own sake.

Breathing exercise

Stand comfortably, feet apart, before an open window if it is raining or otherwise in a well ventilated room.

Place your hands on the lower part of the rib cage on each side with the fingers pointing forwards and just touching at the tips. Inhale deeply and, as you start to fill the lower lungs, the ribs will expand forcing the hands apart a little. At the commencement of inhalation the diaphragm, the sheet of muscle which separates the chest and the abdomen, descends and forces out the upper abdominal muscles. This is known as abdominal breathing and is practised by singers and actors.

Open the back of the nose as you breathe in and you will become aware of air reaching the sinuses. Imagine the cavities of the sinuses opening to receive life-giving oxygen. Inhale it right to the base of the lungs before filling the upper lungs. Then exhale a little more forcefully depressing the rib cage until you have got all the air out. You need to do this before breathing in again.

Humming

Singing is an excellent way of keeping the sinuses in good shape. The well trained voice is projected from the sinuses and back of the nose. This is why many singers can perform even with a cold. They usually sing above the sensitive throat and the vocal chords which would otherwise quickly become irritated.

The resonance created by the production of the note helps to stimulate the sinuses and keep the surfaces clear of excess mucus. Humming or chanting achieves this equally well. Use every opportunity to hum a happy tune, if you feel so inclined, but you may find the meditator's *ohm* the most convenient and effective way of loosening stuffy sinuses. This is a chant used to concentrate the mind and send beneficial vibrations through the body. (It has nothing to do with the similarly named electrical unit of resistance!)

To perform this useful little exercise inhale deeply through the nose and sinuses then sing 'oh-o-o-mmm', allowing it to trail off into a prolonged hum. Pitch it on a comfortable note in the middle of your vocal range. Chant the ohm in conjunction with your breathing exercises and the benefits will be far reaching.

According to Andre van Lysebeth, author of *Yoga Self Taught* (Allen and Unwin, 1971) the *ohm* not only stimulates the sinus and nasal areas but also the endocrine glands, deeper tissues, and nerve cells, having all-round benefits both physically and mentally.

Breathing effectively is an integral part of the gentler systems of exercise, such as yoga, t'ai chi, and Qi gong.

Yoga

The ancient Indian exercise system of yoga not only increases physical mobility but has a reintegrating effect on the whole body. Basically it is a series of 'postures' or *asanas* which are gentle rhythmical movements. The breathing exercise I have described is based on yoga principles which are primarily concerned with promoting the 'life force' or *prana* in the body.

The yoga method of breathing is known as *pranayama* and there are other aspects to the system, such as the physical exercises (*hatha yoga*), and relaxation, all designed to restore internal equilibrium.

Dr Robin Monro, of the Yoga Biomedical Trust, in Cambridge, conducted a survey among three thousand people who practise yoga regularly. Of 226 with asthma and bronchitis, 88 per cent claimed that they had received positive benefit by doing yoga.

There are many yoga postures and it would be wise to learn them in a class where you can be guided by an experienced teacher in the correct way to do them. There is, however, one sequence of movement which is a supreme method of reintegrating the body and loosening up many joints and muscles. It need only take ten minutes first thing in the morning and is an invigorating start to the day. It is called, most appropriately, Salutation to the Sun. It opens the airways wonderfully.

Salutation to the Sun

Wear loose or comfortable clothing. Shorts, track-suits, pyjamas or, if warm enough, nakedness are equally suitable.

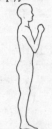

(a) breathe out

1. Stand with bare feet firmly on the floor about nine inches apart, knees very slightly bent, body upright but comfortably poised with neck and shoulders relaxed. Face the east if possible, and exercise before an open window if you are indoors.

2. Place the palms of the hands together in front of the chest with your elbows forward so that the wrists are at right angles. Breathe out slowly.

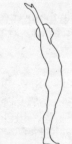

(b) breathe in

3. As you breathe in again (remember to open the sinuses) link your thumbs and turn the palms of the hands to the front. Stretch the arms and hands forwards and up over your head, then lean back as far as you can comfortably go.

(c) breathe out

4. Now bend forwards with the arms outstretched and reach towards your toes, breathing out as you do so. You don't need to keep the legs straight, nor is it necessary to reach the floor if you are not supple enough. Just bend over as far as you can with the head tucked under towards your knees.

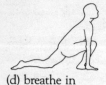

(d) breathe in

5. Next stretch your left foot and leg out behind you along the floor while you bend the right knee and place your hands on the floor in front of you. Stretch your arms and bend the head back as you breathe in. This should become one smooth movement.

(e) hold

6. Bring the right foot back level with the left, bend the head forward and push your bottom up into the air. You are now in an inverted 'V'. This movement is done fairly quickly while you hold your breath.

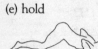

(f) breathe out

7. Breathe out as you bend your arms and lower your body until your toes, knees, chest, and forehead are touching the floor.

(g) breathe in

8. Breathe in again as you stretch the arms, pushing your head and shoulders back, arching the back but with the legs and feet still contacting the floor.

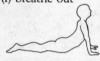

(h) breathe out

9. Draw the feet up so that you are in the inverted 'V' position again, breathing out as you do it.

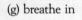

(i) breathe in

10. Now bring the left foot up beneath your chest keeping the right stretched out behind you, bending back neck and shoulders as you breathe in.

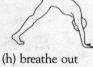

(j) breathe out

11. Draw the right foot up beside the left to bring you into the bent double position again. Breathe out while you do this.

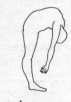

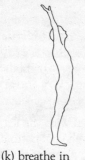

12. Breathe in again as you straighten up and bend back with arms over the head.

(k) breathe in

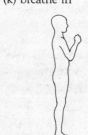

13. Return to the starting position with the hands in the prayer attitude again. You can repeat the sequence or relax the arms to the standing position.

(l) breathe out

Figure 13. 'Salutation to the Sun'.

T'ai chi and qi gong

The Chinese, too, have an ancient system of breathing and exercise devised to improve the flow of the body energy, which they call Chi or Qi (pronounced chee). Every morning the parks, squares, and open spaces in China are filled with people performing a sequence of slow rhythmical movements, known as T'ai chi. The movements are closely related to the breathing and need to be learned correctly and in the right order.

Another Chinese system of exercise, which also imparts great benefit to the lungs and sinuses, is Qi gong, in which the movements are based on those of animals and birds, such as the Crane.

Classes in T'ai chi and Qi gong are held at various centres and it will be well worth the effort of joining one to add either one of these techniques, or yoga, to your armamentarium against hay fever.

Rest and sleep

While we are awake and active, physically or mentally, our levels of destructive or catabolic hormones, such as cortisol and catecholamines, remain high. These are the chemicals the body uses to initiate the breakdown of proteins and mobilization of energy reserves. If we produce too many of them, through being overactive or frequently aroused, the energy reserves begin to fall and resistance weakens. The person who is chronically fatigued is, therefore, much more prone to allergic reactions.

During sleep the balance of the body's functions shifts to anabolism — the building of reserves by cell division and protein synthesis. Cortisol levels become lower and deep sleep is the stimulus for the release of growth hormone which encourages the build-up of protein reserves and mobilizes the fatty acids in the body to provide more energy. It is also known that damaged tissues heal more quickly during sleep, so inflamed mucous surfaces in the eyes, nose, and sinuses, are given an opportunity to regenerate.

During a normal night's slumber we pass through different levels of consciousness. These have been monitored in numerous experiments in which volunteers have slept with electrodes taped all over their heads to measure the electrical activity of the brain. These electro-encephalographic (EEG) readings show that there are different cycles of brain activity, each of which appears to play an important role in our processes of regeneration and readjustment. As we fall asleep the amplitude of brain waves slowly becomes greater and we experience vague images and occasional muscle twitches. Within twenty or thirty minutes we sink into a stage of large slow brain waves eventually reaching a deep sleep in which hormonal activity is greatest with higher levels of, for example, the growth hormone. Deep, stage IV, sleep occurs mostly in the early hours of the morning, so the old maxim about an hour's sleep before midnight being worth two after it has some validity.

If you have difficulty in sleeping, a herbal sedative, such as Passion Flower (*Passiflora incarnata*) may help. To draw the blood away from an overactive mind that hinders sleep, bathe the feet and legs in cold water for two minutes then dry with a rough towel before retiring to bed.

12 *Clearing the Air*

Filters, ionizers, and a big bubble

So far in this handbook we have explored the ways of making our bodies more resistant and alleviating their streaming, stuffy, and irritating symptoms, but what about changing our surroundings? Is it possible to create an atmosphere in which to live and work that is free of pollens and other annoying particles? It would be virtually impossible to do this without creating an artificial environment and losing many of the health advantages of our natural habitat, but a number of devices have been invented to reduce the level of the impurities in the air we breathe.

There are, of course, no substitutes or short-cuts when it comes to health, and the first priority must be to get our own bodies in better working order, but if the intensity of exposure to external irritants can be reduced it all helps to slow down the rate of progress from allergic reaction to acute symptoms (see Figure 14).

Air pollution

A major concern of industrialized and automated societies is the rising level of atmospheric pollution. Fumes from factories, cars, and chemicals in the home, add to the total toxin load the body has to deal with.

Synthetic products, increasingly a part of the home and work environment may induce rhinitis or nasal irritation. Formaldehyde, for example, is present in the glue used to make hardboard, or chipboard. The air of newly built homes may have a high formaldehyde

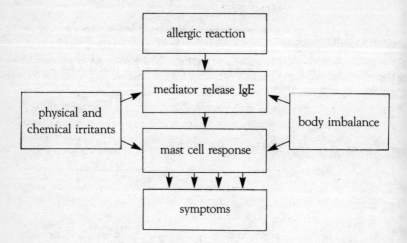

Figure 14. Extra irritants intensify hay fever symptoms.

concentration. Only age and good ventilation reduces the level of formaldehyde in the air of these dwellings. Sulphur dioxide from industrial fumes, will reduce the efficiency of the cilia of the mucous membranes, hindering their task of removing pollen particles, fungal spores, and surplus mucus from the nose, sinuses, and lungs.

The intensity of the reaction to pollens in the hay fever season will be greater in the person who is exposed to other irritants such as house dust, smoke, and industrial fumes. According to Dr J.T. Connell, writing in the *New York State Journal of Medicine* in 1970, the hay fever patient in the pollen season reacts to an allergic dose fifty times lower than that needed to elicit symptoms before the season. Once sensitized the heightened reactivity to such things as house dust or animal dander continues for some weeks.

You can reduce the allergen load of your home environment by regular cleaning of carpets and furnishings. The house dust mite may be curtailed by covering matresses with plastic sheets and will be destroyed by temperatures below 50°F (10°C). Dr Caroline Shreeve, in the *New Era Guide to Hay Fever* (leaflet available from health food stores) recommends deep-freezing pillows in rotation, allowing time for them to thaw out before use!

Smoking

Apart from the well-known hazards to the health of the smoker, second-hand smoke has been shown to convey most of the same disadvantages to other people in the same room. Among these are significant losses of vitamin C and a higher incidence of respiratory ailments. Smokers lose up to 25mg of vitamin C with every cigarette they smoke and non-smokers, breathing the same polluted air, suffer losses of this important vitamin to nearly the same degree.

Nicotine also has an adverse effect on blood-sugar levels, thereby increasing the allergic tendency. The message is clear — if you have hay fever keep away from smoke.

Clearing the air you breathe may reduce the allergic sensitivity and air filters, ionizers, humidifiers, and a space age helmet are among the equipment which may help to relieve your hay fever.

Air scrubbers

Most people spend the majority of their time indoors, even in the summer pollen season, so it is relatively easy to take steps to control the particles in the air they breathe. The idea of 'scrubbing' the air clean of cigarette smoke, motor fumes, and dust particles, may seem far fetched but it is at least possible to reduce the concentration of these pollutants in the air by filtering them out electrostatically.

Many of the particles which are a threat to health are under ten microns in diameter. Pollen grains range in size from under ten to over thirty microns, but fungal spores may be three to five microns in diameter. Cigarette smoke particles are one micron and, therefore, much more likely to be absorbed and contribute to internal irritation. Most filters used in air conditioning systems are inefficient at removing many of these particles, but the Israeli manufacturers of the Amcor Air Processor claim that their equipment is capable of significantly reducing these pollutants. The Air Processor is combined with an ionization unit and this may account for its greater ability to clear finer particles from the atmosphere.

Ionizers

Ions are electrically charged molecules of carbon dioxide, nitrogen, and oxygen which occur naturally in the air. They may be either positively charged or negatively charged, the amount of each changing according to the atmospheric conditions. Positively charged ions predominate in built up areas, heavy traffic, in rooms with electronic equipment, such as computers, video recorders, T.V. sets, and wherever there are high levels of atmospheric pollutants.

Ion levels rise before a thunderstorm, with more positive ions, but after the storm the negative ions predominate. Levels of negative ions are also much higher near waterfalls (formed by the splitting of water droplets), in mountainous regions, and beside the sea. They are believed to be beneficial to health in a number of ways and they may be one reason for the relief the hay fever sufferer gets at the seaside.

Ionizers are electrical devices which produce ions artificially by passing a current to a needle of thin wire which attracts the positive ions and emits the negative ones in a fine stream which can sometimes be felt close to the machine as an 'ion breeze'. Some models use a carbon filament instead of needles to generate the ions.

Scientific tests have shown that negative ions help to reduce smoke, dust, soot, pollens, and bacteria, by attaching themselves to the particles and attracting them to the ground.

Negative ions for hay fever

Whether negative ions have a positive benefit on bodily health or whether they simply settle pernicious particles and make the air better to breathe is a matter for conjecture. Among the health benefits reported are increased vital capacity, an increase of ciliary activity, reduction of blood pressure, reduction of serotonin (a neuro-hormone which plays a part in the onset of pain and inflammation), and a reduction of blood histamine levels. Dr Felix Sulman of Jerusalem, reported a 50 per cent fall in blood histamine levels in a group of patients after regular exposure to negative ions.

A study of the effect of negative ions on hay fever was carried out in the late 1950s by Dr I.H. Kornblueh and colleagues at the North East General Hospital, Philadelphia. Of 123 patients there were 74 who had moderate to severe pollinosis immediately before exposure to ionization. They formed a group who were unknowingly allowed to breathe air with either high negative ions, predominently positive ions, or normal air. Out of the 54 exposed to negative ions 34 (62.9 per cent) reported partial or complete relief of their hay fever. A second group of 49 had a history of hay fever but no current symptoms and were subdivided for exposure to different air conditions in the same way as the first group. All of the 37 cases exposed to negative ions remained free of reactions, whereas a recurrence of acute symptoms was observed in 6 out of 10 of those exposed to positive ions. Of the 2 remaining patients in a normal atmosphere one had a relapse (see Figure 15).

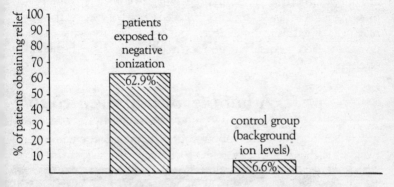

Figure 15. Relief from symptoms of hay fever in 54 cases exposed to negative ions.

Choosing an ionizer

A number of makes of ionizer are on the market and can be obtained from health food stores, chemists, or department stores. All reputable brands are tested and guaranteed for electrical safety and negative ion output. Some have ion indicators to show when they are producing negative ions.

Standard models are portable, some battery operated, and are suitable for a small room, but you will need a more powerful one for bigger offices or rooms where there is much smoke or a lot of electrical equipment. Some manufacturers combine the ionizer with an air filter. Obviously these cannot process all the air in a room so they should be placed on a reasonably high surface, such as a desk or filing cabinet, to ensure that the ions are concentrated in the air you breathe. The maximum ion concentration is about 4-6 feet from standard models and this is a suitable distance for an ionizer in the bedroom.

Models suitable for use in a car are made by Amcor, Medion, and

Mountain Breeze. Car ionizers are generally plugged into the lighter socket.

Humidity and humidifiers

Warm moist air improves the symptoms of hay fever but most centrally heated houses and offices tend to have too dry an atmosphere. This may encourage more dust and pollen movement in the air. A humidifier, or even a bowl of water in the room, may overcome this to some degree but controlled trials have shown no specific effect on nasal function as a result of changes in the humidity of clean air.

A bubble for hay fever trouble

If you can't control the purity of the air in your general surroundings, what about your own immediate environment? Designer Richard Hinchcliffe, himself a hay fever victim for many years,

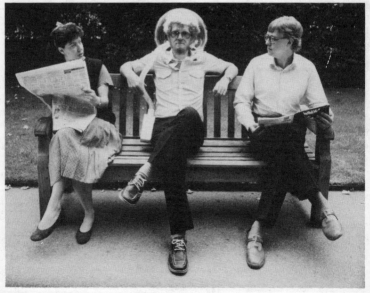

The hay fever helmet — everyday wear or a last resort?

(Photography courtesy of *Which?* magazine)

decided to create his own clean air bubble. He invented the Hincherton Hay Fever Helmet, a clear plastic dome into which filtered air is pumped at low pressure.

The helmet is supported by shoulder braces and air is pumped into the back through a flexible tube connected to the filter pack which is strapped to the waist. The battery, filter pack, and helmet weigh 4 lbs.

The helmet can be worn for periods of 20-30 minutes several times a day, for example, in the morning or evening, or while cutting the lawn. The more audacious can even wear it to work! Breathing clear air for a time allows the mucous membranes to recover some resistance.

The makers claim that over 80 per cent of hay fever users of the helmet found it helpful and some said that they remained symptom-free for several hours after wearing it.

13 *Subtle Energies*

Getting the body back in tune

Most medical treatments, and many of the natural measures I have described here, are based on our knowledge of the anatomy and physiology of the body. We still have much to learn about the intricate workings of our immune system and quite often the most carefully conceived treatment regimen fails to make life for the hay fever sufferer sufficiently tolerable. In such circumstances we cannot afford to ignore the influence upon our health of the even more complex electromagnetic forces to which we are subject.

Surrounding and within our bodies is a sophisticated system of subtle energies, no less important to our well-being than the biochemical factors which we can analyse and measure. That energy forces affect our health has been known to mankind for many thousands of years. When the Chinese evolved their system of medicine, including acupuncture, they developed a concept of energy, or *chi*, within the body which governs its response to the external environment and regulates the internal functions to maintain health. The Indian yoga system of exercise and meditation was devised to restore harmony to a number of major energy centres, the *chakras*, which in turn help to maintain our physical and emotional comfort.

Through the centuries healers of many kinds have utilized these energies, either knowingly, or unknowingly, to help sick people. For many years the idea that there was anything more than the skin and bones, and cells and blood, which can be seen, felt, or measured, was totally discredited by science, but now, in the late twentieth century, the development of electronic instruments which can detect and register these subtle energy forces in the body has brought us to the brink of a fascinating new era in health care. This revival of the wisdom of the ancient physicians has been the spur to the medicine of the future — a subtle and gentle medicine in which the disharmonies of our bodies may be detected and corrected even before they manifest themselves as physical symptoms.

Body rhythms

Many physical functions of the body are at the mercy of the rhythmical fluctuations of energetic forces. Levels of hormones, such as cortisol, vary at different times of the day. You may have noticed that the intensity of your hay fever symptoms is much less on certain days even though you may have made no attempt to control the symptoms, and the pollen count remains high. These variations in our ability to cope with health problems are due, in part, to changes in the rhythm of body cycles — the biorhythms.

From the moment of our birth our body has three distinct cycles of function — a physical cycle of 23 days, an emotional cycle of 28 days, and an intellectual cycle of 33 days. According to biorhythm theory each cycle has a positive and negative phase. In the positive phase our performance is at its best and in the negative phase we are likely to be more sensitive and susceptible to illness. Days when two or more rhythms cross over are said to be critical days when we may be vulnerable in various ways.

It is possible to check your cycles using a biorhythm calculator which is sold by some health food stores. If low physical cycle phases or critical days coincide with rising pollen levels you should take extra care to avoid excessive exposure. You can also anticipate low physical and emotional phases by boosting your intake of protective nutrients and health-promoting herbs.

Geopathic stress

For some sensitive individuals the electromagnetic forces of their immediate surroundings can be a source of interference with the natural process of recovery. An energetic influence relating to the living or working environment can so disturb the body's subtle electromagnetic fields that otherwise beneficial treatments fail to bring more than moderate improvement. Such interference may be due to geological factors or geographical position and is, therefore, called *geopathic stress*. This is clearly an important influence on our health which we are only just beginning to understand.

Geopathic stress can be caused by mineral deposits, certain buildings, movement of underground water, and ley lines, the grid lines of electromagnetic force around the earth. The ley lines are believed to be responsible for cyclical illnesses, those which occur in a regular sequence. Like the tides, they are affected by the lunar cycles, expanding their range of influence at the time of the full moon.

If your hay fever appears to be worse in certain areas and you cannot account for it by differences in the likely levels of pollens or the plants from which they derive, geopathic factors may be responsible. Sometimes these can be determined by using some of the subtle energy techniques of diagnosis about to be described. In the severest cases a change of home or workplace may be necessary to escape the disturbance, but most influences of this sort can be dealt with by less dramatic measures and, before contemplating any such move, you should obtain careful professional advice from a practitioner capable of determining the relevance of such influences on your health.

The body as a computer

Throughout our lives all that we experience is recorded by our body. Much of it — insignificant events, mild scrapes, or minor infections which are happily resolved — is wiped off the tape. Others — physical injuries, emotional shocks, suppressed fevers — may be retained and stored, whether by the brain, nervous system, or energy fields of the body is not clear, but it can be recalled in much the same way as we obtain information from a computer.

A great deal of the material that we retain is filed away harmlessly, but some of it can be a constant depressant of normal immunity if unidentified and unresolved. Gradually, however, we are learning to tune into this information locked in our bodies. By the use of such methods of diagnosis and treatment as radionics, radiesthesia, clinical kinesiology, and bioelectronic instruments, it is becoming possible to retrieve information from each person's body about the individual state of health at ultra-fine levels.

Very often the body hides the information it is storing by making an adjustment or a false adaptation to prevent the toxic factor or injury from causing major disturbance. These factors can, however, insidiously undermine the health if they are not adequately neutralized. The principle of diagnosis using subtle energy techniques is to encourage the body to yield the information again, by testing muscles, or points which indicate the state of the part being investigated. While many sophisticated instruments are being developed for this purpose one of the most effective ways of eliciting information is by testing the muscles of the patient.

Muscle indicators

The intricate interconnections between the different parts of the body are such that the strength of certain muscles can be affected by any changes in the function of body tissues. This principle was discovered by an American chiropractor, Dr George Goodheart, who developed the system of *Applied Kinesiology*. Kinesiology is the science of muscle activation and balancing. Goodheart's system utilizes modern nerve physiology with eastern energy theories to check areas of strength and weakness in body function. It is based on the simple principle that certain muscles become weak when there is a disturbance or interference in the body's electromagnetic field.

Muscles which are tested in this way are called 'indicator muscles', for example, the deltoid muscle which raises the arm above the head is often used. With the patient sitting or lying, an arm is raised straight out in front, with the elbow locked straight. The operator attempts to push the arm down while he makes contact with the area or organ under suspicion with the other hand, touching special energy points, or the skin over the organ. In normal health the patient can resist the pressure on the outstretched arm, but the indicator muscle weakens if there is deficiency or disturbance in the area under test.

This method may also be used to test for sensitivities to foods and other toxins which cause an indicator muscle to weaken when they are brought into the body's electromagnetic field by placing a small morsel on the tongue or over the abdomen.

Applied Kinesiology, and its more recent refinement Clinical Kinesiology, is now used by many practitioners to determine allergic tendencies, and, more importantly, the imbalances which cause them.

It is a technique which is still being evolved and requires a thorough knowledge of anatomy and physiology to be used effectively. It is essential to ensure accuracy in testing of muscle groups as errors can readily arise over foods or other substances to which you may be sensitive.

A simplified layman's version of Applied Kinesiology is taught, called Touch for Health, in which some basic muscle tests and correction procedures can be used.

Tuning in to body waves

When we switch on our radio set we use the power of the battery or electricity to tune in to a wavelength on which we can receive the broadcast sound. We can see or feel nothing but we are able to hear voices or music transmitted from many miles away. Radionics uses much the same principle to tune in to the body's vibrations. Just as we use the selector knob on our radio to pick up different stations, so a radionic practitioner can use an instrument which receives impulses from the body with which it is connected, either physically, through an electrode, or through electromagnetic waves, using a sample from the patient, such as a blood spot, saliva, or hair. The sample, or 'witness', carries the resonance with that individual's energies.

Radionics often involves the use of instruments which concentrate the energy field, whereas radiesthesia makes more use of the dowsing principle in which the sensitivity of the operator is concentrated through a pendulum to receive the information about the patient. Changes in the rhythmical swing of the pendulum over the sample can, in the hands of an experienced dowser, yield information about the health of the patient in a similar way to the muscle tests of applied kinesiology.

A dual harmony

The success of the radionic diagnosis and treatment depends on the practitioner getting into harmony with the patient's energy in order to be able to detect its changes. This is often achieved with the aid of the instrument.

A radionic instrument can appear rather daunting at first sight. Some models have a control panel with a mass of knobs with which the practitioner tunes to the different aspects of bodily function. The patient sits beside the machine and is connected to it, either by holding an electrode or by means of a metal plate placed against the solar plexus, just below the ribs. This merely enables the machine to register the resonance of the patient; there is no sensation at any time. The practitioner must then tune the machine to his own resonance and to that of the patient before testing the vitality of different organs and tissues in the body. The practitioner is an important part of the circuit because the readings are determined by tuning the machine until there is no longer any resistance when he rubs his fingers over a special smooth surface of polished wood or tightly stretched rubber on the control panel. All vitality readings are made by comparing them with an established normal level for each type of organ or function so that a low reading would suggest poor vitality or underactivity.

A typical hay fever case tested in this way was a young man of nineteen who showed imbalances in a number of organs. There were reduced vitality readings on the ileum (small intestine), bladder, bronchial tubes, heart muscle, and head of the pancreas. These would be consistent with poor eliminative functions. The test also showed distinct allergic tendencies and sensitivities to a number of foods, including cow's milk, cheese, chocolate, cola drinks, salt, sugar, dates, and white flour pastas. Toxic deposits were revealed, especially in the sinuses, and may have been the residue of old catarrhal infections. Tests of this type can sometimes reveal unexpected weaknesses which may be causal factors in the chain of pathology leading to the actual disorder.

With radionic testing it is possible to identify specific allergens including individual types of pollen to which you may be sensitive. To do this, however, it is necessary to have samples of the grasses from which they derive although some practitioners claim to be able to make a mental connection by, for example, concentrating on the name or an illustration of the plant, which brings it into the circuit. A sensitivity is indicated by a reduction in the reading for tissues which may be affected, such as the nose or conjunctiva of the eyes. Once identified the guilty grasses can be prepared as a homoeopathic remedy. When selecting a remedy, whether a potentized pollen, a herbal medicament, or nutritional supplement, there should be an increase in the vitality reading when it is brought into the circuit indicating that it is appropriate and in harmony with the patient's needs.

This rather lengthy description of a radionic diagnosis has been given because it explains principles which apply to nearly all subtle energy techniques, including applied kinesiology and the more recent developments of bioelectronic regulatory techniques, such as Mora Therapy and Vega Testing. In the hands of experienced practitioners these techniques may offer hope of a precise way of treating hay fever. The wise practitioner concentrates on detecting and treating the imbalances in the body rather than 'allergy testing' which can be open to error.

Some radionic diagnoses and treatment can be done at a distance using a witness to communicate with the patient's energy. Attempts to discredit these techniques by submitting false samples or duplicate specimens, are meaningless because many sensitivities and imbalances are transitory phenomena. Comparisons of the results determined by these methods with skin prick tests for allergies are also futile because the type of sensitivity being registered is quite different. On the other hand, for the same reason, radionic findings of food or other allergens should not be taken too seriously without the advice of the practitioner who should have wide enough clinical experience to place them in a proper perspective.

The Mora method

The Mora is one of the more elaborate pieces of sophisticated electronic equipment, developed in Germany, for both diagnosis and treatment of subtle energy imbalances.

As with many bioelectronic instruments, no electric current is involved. The patient and the machine form a circuit, and the patient's own electromagnetic oscillations are used. Frequencies, whether harmonic or disharmonic, are received by the machine via an electrode. These then undergo filtration and a process of wave inversion before being fed back to the patient. Weakened oscillations may be amplified before feedback. These changed oscillations are said to restore harmonious vibrations within the patient's electromagnetic fields promoting better functional equilibrium.

The Mora can also be used for testing foods or medicines on the radionic principle. There is no sensation when you have tests or treatment with this equipment but the results can often be quite rewarding, particularly in allergic disorders, where treatment of other more basic problems has failed to bring about an improvement.

Vegatest

The Vegatest machine is another bioelectronic instrument which makes fine measurements of body energies and can provide extensive information about the nature of their imbalance. The instrument includes a 'honeycomb', a set of tubes which can hold ampules of any test substance which is brought into the circuit.

A major feature of the Vegatest method is that the body must be stressed to unmask its imbalances. The reasoning behind this is that our self-regulatory mechanisms at the electrical level are very efficient at covering up a toxic focus, such as infected sinuses or bad teeth, so that their effect may not be apparent. The stress is applied by bringing a sample of a known poison, such as the weed killer Paraquat, into the circuit or by giving a brief electrical stimulus to acupoints on the hand. This shakes up the body's energies sufficiently for them to reveal the true vitality readings of the different tissues.

Tests are then made for general vital reserve (sometimes referred to as the biological age), geopathic stress, areas of toxic focus, psychic (emotional) stress, state of the immune system, and so on, checking a whole sequence of factors affecting health, including food sensitivities. As with the radionic method there is a reduction of the reading for each unsuitable substance, or an improvement for remedies or supplements which can help. The Vegatest is complex and, like the other techniques described here, requires the mental concentration of the practitioner to obtain the best results.

Help for hay fever

Just how helpful can these methods of diagnosis be for the hay fever sufferer? Bioelectronic and radionic techniques are tuning in to very fine levels of body function. They are capable of detecting imbalances long before the actual pathology occurs and may, therefore, have a very big role to play in preventive medicine for the future.

Because of this highly refined level of diagnosis, the operation of these methods calls for considerable skill, without which there may be a high degree of error. In experienced hands the bioelectronic techniques are reported to have successfully identified the real causes of illness in over 80 per cent of cases. Information specifically on hay fever is not well documented, but for the long-term management of the condition these methods offer good prospects of identifying and removing basic causes, especially in intractable cases where obscure imbalances may perpetuate the problem. In acute attacks the appropriate homoeopathic or herbal remedy can also be selected with greater accuracy.

Healing

The principle of electromagnetic energy is also used in healing by hand. Healers have traditionally been those who have a gift for mobilizing the patient's self-restorative forces by placing their hands on, or even just close to, the patient's body. It isn't always necessary to have physical contact with the skin; many healers work on the aura, the layer of energy that surrounds all living things. (Strictly speaking the Therapeutic Touch taught by Doris Krieger and referred to in Chapter 10 is not actual touch but is done by working a little way from the surface to calm and rebalance the patient's energy.)

The benefits of healing are general rather than specific, although the body will use it according to its greatest need. Energy can be directed to certain parts of the body, such as the throat or sinuses.

Most of us possess some capacity to heal with our hands, but few people actually allow this faculty to develop. You can start to improve the sensitivity of the hands by rinsing them with cold water whenever you wash them. After drying give the hands a vigorous shakedown to get the circulation and energy into the fingers and then try this little experiment to feel the energy.

Hold the hands up in front of you, palms facing each other. Close your eyes and bring the hands slowly together. Move them apart again and then repeat the process until you feel a slight warmth or sense of resistance as if you were squeezing a balloon. With practice you may be able to move hands wider apart and feel the change in the resistance of the energy.

Having communicated with your own energy you may now be able to use it to help relieve your own or your child's or partner's hay fever. The eyes can be helped by an exercise known as palming.

Place the palms of the hands gently over the closed eyes which should focus on distance to encourage relaxation. Hold the hands in this position for a few minutes to allow the energy of the eyes time for regeneration and to rest them. This will reduce irritation and watering.

The hands may also be placed on or over the forehead, throat, and back of the neck to transmit healing energy and the technique may be combined with the treatment of reflex points using The Hay Fever Reflex Workout (see page 121).

Colour therapy

The colour of our surroundings has an important influence on our well-being, especially emotionally. Blues and greens, for example, are calming, whilst other colours, such as reds, are stimulating. The reason is that another form of healing energy is transmitted by the colours of the visible light spectrum. Practitioners who use colour therapy make use of this principle in treating their patients' subtle energy. Colour filters are used to direct light of selected colours on the patient according to the desired effect.

Hay fever subjects are bathed in colours which reduce inflammation and irritation, such as the blues or greens, which are also astringent and antiseptic. Pale yellow might also be used to encourage skin functions and reduce the stress on the mucous membranes. To promote drainage of the lymphatic system and reduce wheeziness or asthmatic tendencies stronger yellows or orange might be applied. Orange is also beneficial for the more tenacious type of mucus which it helps to loosen.

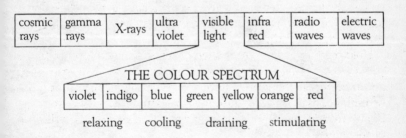

cosmic rays	gamma rays	X-rays	ultra violet	visible light	infra red	radio waves	electric waves

THE COLOUR SPECTRUM

violet	indigo	blue	green	yellow	orange	red

relaxing   cooling   draining   stimulating

Figure 16. Electro-magnetic spectrum.

A hay fever treatment sequence will start with the stronger colours first; for example, the orange, directed mainly to the sinuses or chest for five minutes, followed by ten minutes of yellow to the whole upper body and, finally, blue or green directed to the head or sinus areas to reduce inflammation and promote regeneration.

Some thought may also be given to the colours you wear if your hay fever is particularly troublesome. Thought also can be brought to bear on the problems of hay fever in other ways, and this is covered in the next chapter.

14 *Mind Power*

Thinking a way out of your allergy

To many people the manifestations of the subtle energies are purely products of the imagination. They find it difficult to accept that there is any reality to the electromagnetic forces of the body, even though they cannot deny their effects. Mental faculties of both practitioner and patient are certainly an important element of the diagnostic process in the techniques described in the last chapter but imagination can play an even greater part in the susceptibility to allergy.

The power of the mind can be exercised in both a positive and negative way to influence hay fever, as was convincingly demonstrated by one allergist who found that his patients reacted with increased symptoms to the suggestion of higher pollen counts when he manipulated the figures which were displayed in his clinic, even though the real pollen levels were low.

The mind can play some cruel tricks on the body. It is not only able to switch on symptoms when there is no physical need for them, but it can also undermine the coping ability of the body and translate its own unresolved conflicts and inadequate emotions into physical vulnerabilities. In other words your susceptibility to pollen allergy or other sensitivities can be increased by emotional stresses, and sometimes symptoms can be an expression of an unresolved state of mind.

Fortunately the same mind power which can undermine health can also be directed to work in a positive way to promote it and help in defeating your hay fever.

Psychosomatic illness

The range of illnesses — and there are many — which have their origins in mental conflicts are described as psychosomatic (from *psyche* = mind, and *soma* = body). They are the product of our body's inability to deal adequately with emotional stress.

Stress is something we are all equipped to cope with. It is the stimulus to the adaptation syndrome in our physical bodies — the inhalation of pollen is a physical stress which precipitates the exaggerated defensive response. But, just as inadequately cleared physical ailments can leave a toxic residue which may slowly grind down our health for years to come, so may unresolved stresses become such a mental millstone that they are converted into physical symptoms. They can be produced by either a single shocking experience or a more prolonged disagreeable strain.

The respiratory system is particularly susceptible to the vicissitudes of our emotional life from a very early age. The unresolved stresses of our early life are often responsible for disturbances of the throat, nose, and chest. Some psychotherapists believe they may even occur at the time of birth or before. The classical psychoanalyst's interpretation of asthma, for example, is that it is a suppressed cry for the mother, many adult asthmatics having been found, in analysis, to have had an early childhood deprived of adequate maternal love. The subconscious restraint of the natural desire to cry out for help or affection translates into a restriction of the outward breath with which the asthmatics are troubled.

Suppressed grief

A similar pattern of mind/body interaction has been postulated by Peter M. Goldman, N.D., D.O., M.B.N.O.A., Director of the College of Psychotherapeutics at Speldhurst in Kent. He suggests that the streaming symptoms of hay fever may be due to an underlying grief. The individual is quite literally crying, perhaps because of some unhappiness which was not adequately expressed in the past.

This does not mean that every case of hay fever is due to suppressed grief, but a few cases who may have failed to respond to reasonable physical measures, such as dietary changes, herbal, homoeopathic, or other natural treatment, could be harbouring subconscious regrets about past events which are simply triggered off by the physical stimulus of the pollens invading the mucous membranes.

There are often emotional and physical susceptibilities existing in the allergic individual at the same time. Psychologists call this the 'summation of stimuli', which is rather like the total life burden referred to on page 25. Symptoms in these people can be precipitated by an emotional or a physical triggering factor.

Facing up to life

Peter Goldman also sees allergic individuals as people who may be in conflict with their environment — often a conflict in which they perceive themselves as the losers. They develop a sense of 'preciousness' or fragility, and may have a subconscious need to cry because of their insecurity and inability to face the challenges of life.

Often the conflicts can be resolved by expressing the suppressed emotions or undertaking challenges, such as physical work, or active hobbies, especially outdoor ones like mountaineering, which satisfy the deep need for adventure.

Many of these theories have still to be put to the test but, if Peter Goldman is right, perhaps we shall soon be able to distinguish the more or less allergic individuals by their characteristics as 'life deniers' or 'life affirmers' determined in a survey carried out by Dr Clive Wood M.Sc., D.Phil., of the Department of Human Sciences, Oxford University, and described in the *Journal of the Royal Society of Medicine*.

Those who 'say yes to life' are described as being predominantly sociable, happy, optimistic, vigorous, and with plenty of drive. The life deniers have poor coping ability, are unsociable, pessimistic, and unhappy. Of course, if hay fever victims are mainly life deniers the question which must be asked is do these characteristics come before the illness or because of it?

The lesson for you is really that, whichever type you may be, the positive affirmation approach can achieve changes in physical well-being.

Mind motivation

Using the mind to motivate the body has always been considered a theoretical probability but only in recent years has it been possible to demonstrate distinct physiological changes as a result of thought processes. It has, for example, been shown that regularly practised meditation and relaxation techniques can lower the blood pressure. This effect can be attributed to the release of physical and mental tension which is obtained whilst meditating, but it is also possible to potentiate defensive processes by positive thought.

Dr Carl Simonton, and his wife Stephanie, a psychologist, have developed a technique for cancer patients which you can apply to boost your defences against hay fever. Using *visualization*, in which the patient spends some time each day imagining the body defences overcoming the tumour, they have been able to prolong the lives of cancer patients significantly when compared to those who did not visualize. It was also found that an increase in the count of defensive white blood cells followed periods of visualization.

The Simonton's method, which is described in their book *Getting Well Again* (Bantam Books, New York 1980), involves conjuring up an image appropriate to the individual and the treatment he is taking. Children might picture an army of jolly dwarfs moving in and clearing away the unhealthy tissues or a sports fan might imagine the tumour cells as the opposing team being roundly defeated by the white blood cells.

You can easily adapt visualization to the treatment of your hay fever.

Visualization Exercise

Spend ten or fifteen minutes once or twice a day lying or sitting quietly with your eyes closed (this approach can be used in conjunction with the relaxation technique described on page 158). Concentrate the mind on the defences of your mucous membrane being sealed up and reinforced to form an impenetrable barrier to the invading allergens. Imagine the cells of your immune system marshalling themselves in defence. Picture the nutritional supplements or the herbs you are taking as an army of cleaners, moving in to cool the inflamed tissues and clearing away the excess histamine.

Auto-suggestion

The visualization method is really a form of auto-suggestion. Auto-suggestion was originated by a French apothecary,

Emile Coué, who coined the phrase 'every day, in every way, I am getting better and better'. Although it may sound corny, the work of the Simontons and others has shown that positive affirmation of this sort can bring definite physical benefits.

Autogenic training makes use of the principles of auto-suggestion using simple exercises to induce relaxation which can incorporate the use of autogenic phrases — positive affirmations of health repeated over and over again. Actually verbalizing such sentences as 'I am no longer sensitive to pollens', or 'My nose and eyes feel cool and comfortable', may concentrate the mind which will then send suggestions through to the physical body.

Hypnotherapy

For those who find it difficult to concentrate their minds on any form of mental imagery, hypnotherapy may provide a suitable alternative. Here the suggestion is made by the therapist while the patient is in a receptive state of mind.

Having established a rapport with the patient, and after determining if she is a suitable subject for hypnosis, the therapist places her in a trance, which is a state of dissociation from reality. This temporarily prevents rational thoughts intruding on the mind and inhibiting the power of positive suggestion.

Hypnotherapists, after suggesting to their patients that they have natural immunity, are able to demonstrate to them that they are not sensitive to pollens by actually exposing them to plants which would normally induce symptoms. The relief may be temporary but it is a valuable part of a programme incorporating physical approaches, such as diet control and herbs or homoeopathy, and, above all, establishes in the mind of the patient that recovery is possible.

The hypnotic trance may also be used to create a more relaxed state in which the therapist can use psychological methods to explore the patient's emotional conflicts.

Learning to let go

The simple ability to relax physically and mentally is something many people have lost. As a consequence they carry around unnecessary muscle tensions and postural stresses, which can interfere with healthy body function, and maintain a high level of arousal, which makes excessive demands on vitality.

There are many similar methods of relaxation which are part of such systems as yoga, but one of the simplest is that evolved by L.E. Eeman, whose methods were based on the polarity of electromagnetic forces in the body and are similar to the more recent autogenic training.

The Eeman Technique is used by many naturopaths to reduce physical tensions in their patients, and it helps them to explore psychological factors. It forms the basis of the system of relaxation which is described here. Regular practice will train your body to wind down from the high stress levels of most day-to-day living and will create that much needed opportunity for healing and regenerative processes to operate. You may find you can enter stage 1 sleep, when levels of destructive hormones are reduced, and the routine is certainly a useful prelude to normal sleep when you settle down at night.

A Relaxation Routine

Object	Complete relaxation of voluntary muscles to enable reduction of waste products produced by their activity, and to reduce oxygen demands. Physical relaxation promotes mental calm.
Time required	Five to ten minutes minimum, or as a preliminary to night sleep.
Place	Anywhere you can lie flat comfortably.
How to relax	(Until you are familiar with the routine, try to get a friend to read this through while you follow it.)

Remove shoes and loosen tight clothing. Lie on your back on a comfortable surface. A small cushion or pillow may support the neck and head.

Lay your hands across your abdomen, with the fingers lightly interlaced, and arms resting on the bed.

Breathe in deeply, filling the abdomen first (diaphragmatic breathing), and then sigh out and repeat this a few times, audibly if it helps.

Now allow the breathing to continue at its own pace and depth, but, as you sigh out, concentrate on one part of your body, letting go with each breath. Start with the ankles and feet, letting them flop outwards where gravity takes them. Feel the joints loosening.

Move on to the legs for the next breath or two, and work up your body, conveying the idea of letting go, as you come to each part, even if it won't quite relax as well as you would like it to.

Once you feel that ankles, legs, and knees are relaxed, forget them and move up in this order:

- hips and thighs — think particularly of the inner thigh muscles, which are often tense as a subconscious protector of the genital organs;
- hands and forearms — feel the small muscles and joints in the fingers relaxing;
- abdomen — let it sag;
- chest — feel the muscles between the ribs letting go;
- the whole back, from the buttocks up to the shoulders — feel them sinking and spreading on the bed;
- neck and shoulders — often difficult to let go but send the message through and it will eventually get there;
- head and face — feel the eyes sinking back into their sockets, jaw muscles slacken, mouth may fall open.

With one or two deeper breaths and sighs feel the whole body sinking into deeper relaxation — sigh ... sink ... and sag.

Your friend can test your relaxation by rolling your legs, or lifting up an arm and letting it drop. You won't hurt yourself if you are quite relaxed.

When you are really floppy just lie and think of green countryside and a blue sky — the colours which aid relaxation. Let your breathing proceed at its own pace; it will sometimes slow right down, or occasionally a deeper sigh will want to come through. Allow any muscular twitches and jerks to take their course. They are just due to tension being released.

Rest for a while like this and you may even fall asleep.

Before you rise Remember the cat; it never leaps up unless it is disturbed. It stretches, a little at a time, to gradually increase the circulation to the muscles ready for more action. You should try to do the same.

Stretch your arms and legs, and breathe a little more deeply, to get the muscles into action, and circulate the oxygen. You will now feel more rested with improved circulation and better energy.

Bach flower remedies

The subtle psychological powers of a selection of flowers were discovered in the 1930s by Dr Edward Bach. He found that the essences of thirty-eight different species of wild flower had a positive effect on emotional states, such as anger, fear, impatience, and grief. Mimulus, for example, is helpful to those who experience fear for known reasons — fear of illness, fear of animals, or fear of death — and you can give them the 'quiet courage to face trials and difficulties with equanimity and humour' (T.W. Hyne-Jones in *Dictionary of the Bach Flower Remedies*, Dr Edward Bach Healing Centre, 1977).

There are a number of the Bach remedies which may help the hay fever sufferer, particularly if there is any likelihood of underlying emotional factors holding back progress towards recovery:

Agrimony	For the person who is restless and seeks excitement.
Centaury	Timid type, easily imposed upon. Low vitality and often too tired to try to get well.
Clematis	Listless, withdraws from difficulties. Promotes purposefulness.

Crab Apple	A cleanser for those who feel unclean physically or mentally.
Gorse	Despair and hopelessness. To cultivate hope in chronic illness.
Honeysuckle	Breaks the bonds with the past. For nostalgia and regrets.
Star of Bethlehem	Remedy for grief, delayed shock, or disappointment.
Walnut	Oversensitive types, especially to past events. For the transition stages in life, e.g., teenager at exam time.
Wild Rose	To overcome resignation to illness. For the person who believes he is incurable.

Laughter

Laughter is reputed to have a positive effect on the immune system. This belief was reinforced by Norman Cousins, an adjunct Professor in the Department of Psychiatry and Behavioural Sciences at the University College of Los Angeles School of Medicine, in his book *Anatomy of an Illness* (W.W. Norton, New York 1979), in which he described his experience in overcoming a terminal illness. Having been given the grave prognosis of the physicians he decided he would not resign himself to the sentence of decline and death but, instead, discharged himself from the hospital and prescribed himself a daily diet of Marx Brothers' films.

Whether it was the laughter which brought about his recovery or his positive affirmation and use of large doses of vitamin C it is difficult to be sure. It was probably the whole package, and introducing a good laugh into your daily routine will only do good for your hay fever. If nothing else the resonance will shake up the nasal and sinus cavities and clear the catarrhal congestion a bit and it may, at least, restore a more positive outlook on life.

15 *Professional Options*

Alternative medical care

In addition to the wide range of self-help measures you can use to treat your hay fever there are now many professional skills upon which you can draw for further assistance. The recommendations made in this handbook are, of necessity, fairly general, although widely applicable, but there may be aspects of health, unique to you, which require individual attention.

Practitioners of natural therapeutics are trained to make a careful clinical evaluation of your health and potential for recovery with special reference to their own system of treatment. Each of the professions described in this chapter are complete medical systems offering safe methods of treating the body to restore health. They are alternatives to conventional medicine, as indeed they are to each other, in the sense that they are different in their approach to illness. The natural therapies have a common objective of restoring the normal self-healing mechanisms of the body. They are not necessarily incompatible with conventional medical treatment and are, therefore, increasingly referred to as complementary medicine.

All of the professional associations of the main systems described here — naturopathy, osteopathy, chiropractic, acupuncture, homoeopathy, and medical herbalism — publish registers of qualified practitioner members which are available from their head offices listed under Useful Addresses (see page 184).

Naturopathy

Naturopathic medicine recognizes that health depends equally upon our emotional, structural, and biochemical functions, all of which must be well integrated for us to remain fit. It is based on principles which are fundamental to all natural therapeutic systems and are the essence of the advice given in this book.

The naturopath carries out a standard medical examination but interprets the results of such investigations as blood pressure, stethoscope examinations and blood tests, in terms of the information they reveal about your vital reserve and potential for recovery. He may back up this information with examination of the spine, reflex areas, the use of applied kinesiology techniques, hair analysis for mineral and trace element levels, and iris diagnosis.

Iris diagnosis

Iris diagnosis (iridology) is inspection of the iris of the eye and its surroundings for signs of abnormality in the tissues which have reflex connections with other parts of the body. It is a valuable way of assessing the overall vitality of the individual, the state of organs, such as the skin, lymphatic system, nervous system, and lungs.

A tendency to poor skin function, for example, may be revealed by a darkening of the zone around the edge of the iris, and lymphatic congestion may be suggested by an irregular ring of white flecks just inside this. Iris signs can, in fact, reveal considerable information about the functional state of the body, and some naturopaths, particularly on the Continent, make almost exclusive use of it. The iris is particularly useful as a pointer to underlying disturbances which can be responsible for allergic manifestations.

The typical hay fever case will often show signs of over-irritation of the mucous membranes by white or light deposits in the eyes and signs of lymphatic congestion. The bowel zones may reveal poor tone and distention, indicative of inadequate elimination, which may also account for signs of skin sluggishness. The signs in the iris must, however, be interpreted in the context of a full clinical assessment to be sure of their significance to your health at any particular time. They may often represent only a tendency to particular disorders which might not need specific attention.

Naturopathic treatment and advice may range widely from counselling and relaxation techniques for the anxious or over tense individual, through hydrotherapy and the use of exercise and sunlight, to dietary advice and applied nutrition — the use of controlled intake of food and of vitamin or mineral supplements — for the management of respiratory problems. Programmes of fasting on raw juices or fruit and vegetable diets under the supervision of naturopaths have proved highly effective in reducing many chronic and acute respiratory disorders. Many health problems, however, are due to undernourishment and the naturopath is able to determine the need for a more constructive nutritional approach. Naturopathic medicine is concerned with the health of the whole person, and practitioners can offer valuable specialist guidance to supplement the other measures you may be undertaking for the management of your hay fever.

Qualified naturopaths hold a Diploma in Naturopathy signified by an N.D. after their name. Members of reputable associations are not allowed to advertise individually.

Medical herbalism

The principles of medicinal herbs and some simple recommendations were made in Chapter 7. More specialized advice on the use of herbal medicines is obtainable from a consulting medical herbalist. The medical herbalist is trained to carry out a full examination along similar lines to that of a doctor or naturopath, and, on the basis of this, he may decide upon appropriate combinations of herbs which are given either as liquid extracts, tinctures, or dried herbs from which you may make infusions. The medical herbalist may also use other forms of diagnosis, such as iridology and radionics.

In treating a case of hay fever the herbal practitioner may choose herbs which promote the skin and bowel function in order to relieve the toxic burden on the mucous membranes. His formulae might also include herbs to assist the function of the liver, and will certainly take account of the need for more immediate relief of the irritated mucous membranes by using anti-inflammatory preparations. The medical herbalist will be able to gauge more accurately the combinations and dosage schedules for the longer term management of your hay fever and will adjust the formulations according to the changing phases of your response.

Medical herbalists may also make dietary suggestions and recommend nutritional supplements or enzyme preparations to promote normal digestive functions.

Successful graduates of a full time training in medical herbalism are awarded a Diploma in Phytotherapy (D.Phyt) and Membership of the National Institute of Medical Herbalists (M.N.I.M.H.).

Homoeopathy

Another method of prescribing uses infinitesimal proportions of plant extracts and minerals to support the functions of the respiratory system and reduce acute symptoms. Practitioners of homoeopathy make a careful assessment of the whole patient, paying as much attention to the mental and emotional influences (and such idiosyncracies as taste preferences, thirst, changes of appetite, and susceptibility to weather changes) as to physical signs and symptoms.

The methods of preparation of homoeopathic medicine have been described on page 92 and the prescription of a practitioner may include some of the remedies referred to there, but he also has a range of many hundreds of others to choose from, some of which may be indicated for your particular symptom peculiarities or personality. Most homoeopaths try to select a single remedy which is most appropriate for the patient, but combinations of two or more remedies may be prescribed.

Homoeopathy is also a safe form of treatment for other respiratory infections, such as colds or 'flu, as an alternative to antibiotics. Antibiotics normally suppress the acute symptoms leaving a residue of catarrh which lays the foundation for future respiratory problems or toxic foci. Homoeopathic medicines encourage their resolution without the likelihood of recurrence of long term complications.

Doctors who have completed the postgraduate course at the Royal London Homoeopathic Hospital become Members of the Faculty of Homoeopathy (M.F.Hom.). Other practitioners, who have taken an extended course and examinations in homoeopathy, may belong to the Society of Homoeopaths.

Acupuncture

Acupuncture is part of a system of medicine which originated in China several thousand years ago, in which the human body is seen as a unified organism made up of interdependent systems which are subject to the internal influences of the emotions; fear, anger, joy, and so on, and the external factors of the environment, such as food, climate, and physical phenomena. Using fine needles, a burning herb, or a mild electrical stimulation, the acupuncturist treats points on the body surface which are believed to be interconnected by channels, known as meridians, that have connections by deeper pathways with the organs of the body. Acupuncture treatment is gentle, painless, and, invariably, most relaxing.

Traditional Chinese Medicine is based on the subtle energy principle that there exists in the body a vital force, known as *chi* which maintains a balance between its polarities of yin, the cool, dark, expansive principle, and yang, the hot, light, contractile principle. Allowing for the natural predominance in the male of the yang principle and in the female of the yin principle, there should, in normal health, be a balance between the two.

In Traditional Chinese Medicine hay fever or allergic rhinitis is regarded as a localized yang condition due to the rising up of the heat or 'fire' from the liver and gall bladder. Fine acupuncture needles might be inserted in points on the face and forehead and left in for ten or twenty minutes to disperse the heat and congestion. Points on either side of the nostrils, for example, used in conjunction with points on the hands, will clear nasal or sinus congestion and reduce inflammation. Other points on the trunk and extremities may be used to promote the natural immunity and correct the imbalance of function in the organs, such as the liver, spleen, or lungs, which are considered to be responsible for the disturbed energy pattern.

Pulse and tongue diagnosis

The practitioner of traditional Chinese acupuncture assesses the requirements of his patient by taking a careful case history, doing a general examination, and paying particular attention to the quality of the pulses on each wrist, and signs revealed by observation of the tongue. This information is then integrated to select the appropriate points and method of treatment.

Acupuncture treatment integrates well with other forms of therapy. Dr Willem Khoe, writing in the *American Journal of Acupuncture*, in June 1979, reported a success rate of over 90 per cent in treatment of over 500 cases of rhinitis and hay fever using a combination of acupuncture, homoeopathy, and nutrition.

Modern research has shown that the stimulation of certain acupuncture points promotes the release by the brain of pain-relieving hormones known as encephalins and endorphins. These may have an anti-inflammatory effect which would also account for the benefit derived by hay fever sufferers from this form of treatment.

Qualified practitioners will either hold a Licentiate in Acupuncture (Lic.Ac) or a Bachelor of Acupuncture (B.Ac.) and the designatory letters of the professional association to which they belong. If you consult only a member of one of the associations listed in Useful Addresses (see page 184) you can be sure of adequate professional skills and proper sterilization and safety procedures.

Osteopathy

The neck has important relationships structurally with sinus and nasal functions. Good posture and alignment of the neck and head are essential to proper lymphatic drainage and will affect the efficiency with which the nose and sinuses operate. People with nasal allergies commonly have displacements of bones in the upper part of the neck which may also affect the nerve supply to the respiratory membranes and increase the sensitivity. The influence extends even further; correcting the restriction of the atlas, the top bone of the spinal column, has been found to bring about improvements in blood sugar levels. General osteopathic treatment to the neck and back also promotes the lymphatic drainage and improves the freedom of breathing.

Osteopathy is a system of medicine which concentrates on reintegrating the joints and muscles of the body, particularly those of the head, neck, and back, to restore better mobility. Restrictions in the movement of the back and neck joints, apart from causing local discomfort, can impair the functions of the nerves which pass out between the bones from the spinal cord to supply all the organs of the body. These limitations of mobility also interfere with the normal flow of blood. The objective of the osteopath is to remove such obstacles to promote healthy function.

The osteopath will usually carry out a general examination because he needs to assess the state of your musculo-skeletal system in the context of your total health. In the examination of the spine he will feel carefully for the position and range of movement of the individual bones and the conditions of the muscles and ligaments. This process of exploratory diagnosis becomes the treatment as stiffened and contracted muscle fibres are stretched and ligament tone is rebalanced by special soft tissue massage techniques which most osteopaths use. Joints are gently eased or more specific manipulative procedures are used to release those which are locked in limited mobility.

Cranial osteopathy

Some osteopaths practice a gentle form of reintegration of the bones of the skull known as *Cranial Osteopathy*. The subtle rhythmical movements of the cranial bones work in harmony with the rest of the spinal column to promote the flow of cerebrospinal fluid which nourishes the brain and nervous system.

Cranial osteopathy is of particular value to people with poor drainage of the sinuses for whom it may help to release the congestion created by narrowed appertures which open into the nasal cavity. Cranial osteopathy is very gentle, as the practitioner simply rests the hands lightly on the head feeling for subtle changes of movement in relation to the breathing and using gentle manoeuvres to help rebalance them.

The designatory letters of qualified osteopaths are D.O. and membership of the relevant professional association (e.g. M.B.N.O.A. or M.R.O.).

Chiropractic

Chiropractic is another system of structural reintegration which differs from osteopathy primarily in the techniques used to achieve this. The chiropractor's main objective is to restore nervous equilibrium by correction of displacements of the spinal vertebrae. Many chiropractors now use the sophisticated systems of muscle reflex testing and treatment in applied kinesiology, and may also use other techniques, such as the Chapman reflexes.

Supplementary specialists

There are various other treatments which, although they are not complete medical systems, can be of great benefit to the person with hay fever.

Alexander Technique

F. Matthias Alexander, an Australian actor, was having chronic throat problems and he discovered that these were due to what he called inappropriate 'use of the self'. To correct these problems he developed the Alexander Technique, a system of teaching postural awareness and relaxation. By lying, sitting, standing, and walking more effectively, you will gain better poise and reduce physical and mental tensions as well as improve the functions of the respiratory system.

Teachers of the Alexander Technique undergo a lengthy and rigorous training and give careful instruction to develop your awareness of faulty habit patterns and cultivate newer healthy ones. To be effective the process takes some months but it is a worthwhile and valuable aid to relaxation and more efficient breathing.

Autogenic Training

This is one of a number of methods of learning to relax and let go physically. The subject is taught how to breathe correctly and release physical tensions in different parts of the body. This method can be used in conjunction with other forms of suggestion to reduce the intensity of your nasal and eye irritation.

Reflexology

This is the specialized technique of foot massage originated by Eunice Ingham in the U.S.A. Reflex zones on the feet are gently massaged to improve the energy and function of the whole body. There are special zones connected with the respiratory organs such as the sinuses, upper lymphatic ducts, nose, and lungs. (See page 124.)

Reflexologists are trained to work specifically on the reflex zones of the hands and feet to promote well-being through their connections with the rest of the body.

16 *Taking the Heat Out of Hay Fever*

The fast relief plan

There *is* an answer to hay fever, but it is not a single universal cure. We are all individuals and the reasons our health and resistance breaks down are many and varied. The paths back to health may be equally diverse, and in this book we have explored a number of those which have lead countless sufferers towards freedom from the purgatory of their pollinosis.

Of the many tips I have included there is, therefore, no single panacea. But, by selectively using a combination of approaches you will gradually eradicate the problem of hay fever. When the fire of your acute symptoms is raging, however, you want something to take the heat out quickly. This can be done most effectively by the *Fast Relief Plan* (FRP).

The FRP uses the principles of fasting and controlled diet in conjunction with other supportive measures to give rapid relief in almost all congestive and inflammatory conditions. It has been used, in one form or another, by thousands of hay fever sufferers to alleviate the itching and sneezing in the most acute stages of the condition.

There are a number of benefits from the Fast Relief Plan:

- Rests the digestive tract.
- Promotes the eliminative functions.
- Reduces mucus discharge.
- Clears nasal and sinus congestion.
- Reduces histamine levels.
- Reduces intensity of allergic symptoms.

The FRP can be undertaken by almost anyone. It will give some immediate relief as well as offering longer term improvement. The allergic reaction may continue if there is further exposure to pollens, but the intensity of the symptoms will be greatly reduced. The more completely you follow the FRP the better will be your chances of a quick reduction of your symptoms, but if it is not convenient to do the complete plan you may undertake it with some modifications and still derive benefit. Alternatively, one of the less onerous cleansing programmes in Chapter 5 may be more manageable for you. If you've got a stuffy head, itching eyes, and streaming nose, however, you cannot do better than plunge into the FRP for a few days to cool things down.

The Fast Relief Plan

First day

Begin the fast with a purgative dose of Epsom salts — a teasponful in a pint of warm water first thing in the morning (if you have a particularly sensitive digestive system you should avoid this procedure).

Throughout the rest of the day, at approximately four hour intervals, take one tumblerful of freshly extracted or unsweetened canned or bottled fruit or vegetable juice. Apple and carrot juice are most suitable — the two can be mixed together. Lacto-fermented vegetable juices, such as celery, carrot, or beetroot, available from health food stores, may be used but should be diluted with mineral water.

To satisfy thirst at other times of the day take a small glass of mineral water with a slice of lemon.

Second day

On rising	Glass of hot water with a dessertspoonful of lemon juice or apple cider vinegar.
Breakfast	Apple juice with mineral water.
Mid-morning	Mineral water with slice of lemon.

Lunchtime	Apple or carrot juice mixture or mineral water.
Mid-afternoon	Herb tea (e.g. chamomile, peppermint, or rosehip).
Evening	Fruit or vegetable juice as before.

Third day

On rising	Herb tea.
Breakfast	Fresh fruit (e.g. apples, grapes, pears, melon, or pineapple, either singly or made into a fruit salad). Plain goat's milk yogurt if desired.
Mid-morning	Mineral water with a slice of lemon.
Lunch	Fresh fruit again.
Evening	Fresh fruit or potassium broth (see page 175).

Fourth day

On rising	Lemon juice with warm water.
Breakfast	Fresh fruit with yogurt.
Mid-morning	Mineral water with lemon.
Lunch	Small mixed salad. Fresh fruit as dessert.
Mid-afternoon	Mineral water with slice of lemon.
Evening	Two or three conservatively cooked vegetables with a baked jacket potato served with a little vegetable oil and cottage cheese.

Fifth day onwards	Continue with the basic outline as above. You may now add some nuts and seeds to the fruit at breakfast and one or two slices of wholemeal bread or toast with a savoury spread.
	Lunch may be expanded to include a savoury dish with the salad or a baked jacket potato.
	The evening meal may consist of a savoury dish with vegetables or mixed vegetable stew. Fresh fruit or natural fruit jelly or a tofu dessert to follow.

| **Supportive measures** | Dry skin brushing or wet friction rub each morning to promote skin function. |

Steam inhalation with a few drops of *Olbas* oil in the water for nasal stuffiness once or twice a day.

Use an ionizer in the bedroom overnight.

Spend ten minutes each morning and evening using a selection of points from the Hay Fever Reflex Workout (see page 120).

Supplements From the third day onwards the following supplements should be taken:

Vitamin A 5,000 IU morning and evening.

Vitamin B complex, 1 daily, full strength.

Vitamin C 500mg (best as bioflavonoids), 2 tablets twice daily (1 twice daily for children).

Zinc orotate 50mg to be taken at night.

Herbal remedies From the third day onwards the following may be taken:

Make an infusion of equal parts of Echinacea (cone flower), Mullein, Elderflower, and Golden Seal.

Take three tablets of Garlic with Fenugreek at night.

Use cold compresses of Eyebright infusion on the eyes when resting.

Use Red sage extract as a gargle — 1 teaspoonful in warm water. (See details of herbal preparations on page 89.)

Homoeopathic medicines Use as an alternative to herbal medicines from the third day onwards. Choose from:

Allium cepa 6 — one tablet every four hours reducing frequency with improvement.

Arsenicum album 6 — one tablet every four hours reducing with improvement.

> *Sabadilla* 6 — one tablet every four hours reducing with improvement.
>
> Biochemic tissue salt *Combination H* — four pilules every three hours.

Note

When you first undertake the FRP there may be an initial aggravation of the symptoms although you should feel somewhat better in yourself. The aggravation may take the form of increased nasal discharge and a loosening of old mucus. This is a natural response to the treatment as the body removes unwanted toxic matter in the form of catarrh.

People with low blood sugar (indicated by feelings of fatigue, headaches, or dizziness when witholding food) should not start with the fast on juices but move straight to the third day, taking fruit and vegetable stew. They should also take a little fruit or some sunflower seeds between the meals.

If you are in any doubt about your ability to undertake this programme you should seek professional advice from a doctor familiar with nutritional treatments, a naturopath, or medical herbalist.

Healthy Recipes for Hay Fever

Starter

Avocado and Cottage Cheese

Ingredients   Avocado pear; cottage cheese; garlic salt; lemon juice.

Method   Mix 2 tablespoons of cottage cheese with a little garlic salt and add a few drops of lemon juice. Halve the avocado pear and remove the stone. Place the cottage cheese mixture in the avocado pear and serve.

Soups

Potassium Broth

Ingredients   2 large potatoes, unpeeled, chopped into approximately half inch pieces; 1 cup carrots shredded or sliced; 1 cup beets shredded and sliced; 1 cup celery, leaves and all, chopped into half inch pieces; 1 cup of any other available vegetables; beet tops, turnips, turnip tops, parsley, cabbage, or a little of everything.

Method   Use stainless steel, enamelled, or earthenware utensils. Fill the utensils with one and a half quarts of water and slice the vegetables directly into the water to prevent oxidation. Cover and cook slowly for at least half an hour. Let stand for another half hour, strain, cool until warm and serve. If not used immediately, keep in the refrigerator. Warm up before serving. Can be used without straining as a stew.

Carrot Soup

Ingredients   2 large carrots; 1 onion; 1 tablespoon wholemeal flour; 2 oz (50g) sunflower oil or margarine (or vegetable oil); 1 teaspoon thyme or other herbs to flavour; 1½ pt (¾ litre) water; sea salt.

Method   Dice carrots; peel and chop onion; sauté in margarine, or oil, with herbs, for 5 minutes. Stir in flour and add water. Cook gently for 30 minutes. Season with sea salt, or add yeast extract to flavour.

Salads

Combination Salad

Ingredients   Half a lettuce; watercress; cress; cucumber; 2 tomatoes; spring onions; 2 medium sized carrots; mint or parsley; milled nuts; lactic or cottage cheese.

Method   Break lettuce into bowl. Add watercress, sliced cucumber, tomatoes, and grated carrots. Garnish with mint and parsley and add spring onions. Sprinkle milled nuts over the salad. Serve with lactic cheese and sunflower oil or salad dressing.

Winter salad

Ingredients   Half head of cabbage; 2-3 medium-sized carrots; half raw beetroot; celery; 1 green pepper; 1 onion; chicory; nuts; raisins; small portion cottage cheese.

Method   Chop or dice the cabbage, celery, pepper, and onion. Grate the carrots and beetroot. Mix all ingredients together in a bowl and add milled nuts and raisins. Break chicory on top and sprinkle dressing over before serving.

Apple and Vegetable Salad

Ingredients   1 apple; celery stalks; lettuce leaves or endive; cucumber; nuts.

Method   Chop the celery, endive, and cucumber. Mix in a bowl rubbed with garlic cloves. Add apple slices and sprinkle with milled nuts. Serve with salad dressing.

Salad dressings

Lemon and Honey Dressing

Ingredients   Corn or sunflower seed oil; pure lemon juice, or apple cider vinegar; 1 teaspoon runny honey; herbs; sea salt.

Method   Mix 75% corn or sunflower seed oil with 25% lemon juice, or cider vinegar, add honey and mix in. Add herbs and sea salt to flavour.

Yogurt Dressing

Ingredients   2-3 tablespoons yogurt; lemon juice; onion or garlic; mixed fresh or dried herbs.

Method   Add frew drops of lemon juice to yogurt and chopped onion or garlic and whisk thoroughly together with mixed herbs.

Tofu Dressing

Ingredients   Half to whole block tofu (200-300g); half cup vegetable oil; 1 tablespoon tamari or soya sauce; 1/3 cup lemon juice; 1 tablespoon tahini; fresh mint leaves.

Method   Place the ingredients in a blender or bowl and chop or break in the mint leaves. Blend or whisk to a thick creamy consistency. May also be used as a dip.

Savoury Dishes

Savoury Grains

Ingredients   Whole cereal grains such as millet, buckwheat, rye, or brown rice may be used as a savoury dish.

Method   Place the grains in a saucepan and just cover with
                water. Bring to boil, replace lid and allow to simmer
                for 5-10 minutes, or longer according to the grain.
                The water should be almost absorbed by the grains.
                Add grated cheese, chopped onions or mushrooms
                and flavour with yeast extracts if desired. Serve with
                salads, or as main dish with 2 or 3 conservatively
                cooked vegetables.

Mushroom and Tomato Savoury

Ingredients   8 oz (225g) breadcrumbs; 8 oz (225g) milled nuts;
                4 tablespoons vegetable oil; 8 oz (225g) mushrooms;
                8 oz (225g) tomatoes; sea salt, herbs to flavour.

Method   Sauté breadcrumbs and milled nuts in vegetable
                oil, stirring frequently until crisp. Chop the
                mushrooms and quarter the tomatoes. Sauté these
                in vegetable oil for 5 minutes. Place a little oil in
                an ovenproof dish and fill with alternate layers of
                the mushroom mixture and the nut mixture,
                adding a little sea salt to each layer, and herbs if
                using. Top layer should be nut and breadcrumb
                mixture. Bake for 30 minutes in a moderate oven.
                Serve with selection of vegetables

Savoury Tofu Flan

Ingredients   Wholewheat pastry 8 oz (225g); tofu 10 oz (280g);
                cooked millet 4 oz (110g); water 8 fl oz (225ml);
                vegetable oil 2 fl oz (50ml); 2 tablespoons tahini;
                2 tablespoons soya sauce; 1 teaspoon brewer's yeast;
                onions (chopped) 8 oz (225g); mushrooms (chop-
                ped) 4 oz (110g); tomatoes (chopped) 4 oz (110g).

Method   Preheat oven to 350°F (177°C) Gas Mark 4. Line
                flan case and bake blind for ten minutes. Sauté
                onions, mushrooms, and tomatoes in a little oil
                until tender. In a blender combine the millet, tofu,
                water, tahini, soya sauce, oil, and brewer's yeast.
                Blend until smooth liquid obtained, mix with
                sautéd vegetables and pour into flan case. Bake for
                40-50 minutes until golden brown.

Desserts

Fruit Compote

Ingredients   Dried apricots; raisins; other fresh fruit in season.

Method   Soak the apricots with the raisins in ½ pt (275ml) of water overnight. Simmer for 15 minutes. Add fresh fruit suitably chopped or grated. Cook for 5 minutes and serve with milled nuts or almond cream. Sweeten with runny honey if desired.

Baked Apple

Ingredients   Large apple; seedless raisins; 2 tablespoons milled nuts.

Method   Core the apple. Fill the centre with raisins. Place in a baking dish in a little water. Bake for 30 minutes. Serve with milled nuts sprinkled on top. Add runny honey to sweeten if desired.

Stuffed Pears

Ingredients   4 pears; almond or cashew cream; 1 tablespoon each of raisins, sliced pineapple, ground walnuts, or almonds.

Method   Halve pears and scoop out cores. Whip almond cream and fold in with raisins, pineapple, and milled nuts and place in the centre of fruit. Serve with runny honey or maple syrup as desired.

Muesli

Method   Soak organically grown crushed oats in water overnight. Approximately 2 cups of water to 1 cup of crushed oats will be required. In the morning add 1 teaspoon pure lemon juice and grated apple and any other fresh or dried fruit as desired. The muesli may be served with molasses, fruit juice, wheatgerm, milled nuts, or almond cream.

Sugar-free Flapjack

Ingredients   Jumbo oats 8 oz (225g); rolled oats 4 oz (110g); wholewheat flour 6 oz (170g); spices to taste; pinch of sea salt; dried fruit 8 oz (225g); roasted nuts 4 oz (110g) (optional); 2 tablespoons honey;

3 tablespoons malt; 10 tablespoons vegetable oil; 6-8 tablespoons water.

Method Mix dry ingredients. Rub in oil and sweeteners. Mix in water and leave for 10 minutes to soak. Bake until golden brown.

Dairy-free Trifle

Jelly Apple juice 1 pint (½ litre); 2 teaspoons agar agar powder.

Cream agar agar in a little cold water and add to warmed apple juice. Simmer for 2-3 minutes.
Place 8-10 wholewheat digestive biscuits in dish. Add 10½ oz (300g) tin drained unsweetened mandarin oranges (or available in natural juice from good supermarkets or health food stores); 15 oz (425g) tin unsweetened drained pineapple pieces, and pour jelly over. Allow to set.

Custard 2½ dessertspoons kuzu (arrowroot will do as alternative); ⅔ pt (375ml) water, or water and fruit juice mixed; 1½ dessertspoons tahini; 1 dessertspoon lemon juice; 2 dessertspoons honey.

Blend the kuzu in a little liquid until smooth. Blend tahini with a little liquid. Heat the rest of the liquid very slowly, adding the kuzu and tahini mixture and stirring until thick and creamy. Add 1 dessertspoon lemon juice and honey to taste, stirring carefully to avoid separation.
Pour the custard over the trifle when jelly is set.

Cashew Nut Cream

Ingredients Cashew nut pieces 3½ oz (100g); tofu 2 oz (55g); water 7 fl oz (200ml); honey 1 teaspoon (optional); 6 drops natural vanilla essence.

Method Roast the cashew nut pieces for 5-7 minutes or until lightly browned. Simmer tofu in water for five minutes. Put cashews into blender and add half of the water. Blend until smooth. Drain tofu and add to blender. Blend, gradually adding the rest of the water. Finally add vanilla essence and honey if required.

Low-fat Frozen Dessert

A quickly made summer dessert as alternative to ice cream.

Ingredients Low-fat natural yogurt 16 oz (500g); half jar sugar-free jam (pure fruit jam) 5 oz (150g); chopped fresh fruit (optional).

Method Blend yogurt and jam thoroughly. Pour into freezer tray and freeze until almost solid. Remove from freezer tray and reblend, adding chopped fruit if desired. Return to freezer to set.

Further Reading

General

Naturopathic Medicine, Roger Newman Turner (Thorsons, 1984)
The Natural Family Doctor, Ed. Andrew Stanway (Century, 1987)

Food

Diets to Help Hay Fever and Asthma, Roger Newman Turner (Thorsons, 1970)
Low Blood Sugar, Martin L. Budd (Thorsons, 1984)
Food Combining for Health, Doris Grant and Jean Joice (Thorsons, 1984)
Nutritional Medicine, Stephen Davies and Alan Stewart (Pan, 1987)

Physical Treatments

Massage at Your Fingertips, (Science of Life Books, 1984)
Massage Therapy, Richard Jackson (Thorsons, 1980)
Healing Massage Techniques, Frances M. Tappen (Reyton Publishing Co. Inc.)
Better Health With Foot Reflexology, Dwight C. Byers (Ingham Publishing Inc.)
Health and Light, John N. Ott (Pocket Books, New York)

Natural Medicines

Herbs for Colds and Flu, Nalda Gosling (Thorsons, 1976)

Healing Power of Pollen, Maurice Hanssen (Thorsons, 1979)
Homoeopathic Medicine, Trevor Smith (Thorsons, 1982)
Dr Schuessler's Biochemistry, J.B. Chapman (Thorsons, 1984)

Exercise

Yoga Self-Taught, Andre van Lysebeth (Allen and Unwin)
Oriental Methods of Mental and Physical Fitness, Pierre Huard and Ming Wong (Funk & Wagnalls, New York)

Mind Power

Getting Well Again, Carl and Stephanie Simonton (Bantam, 1980)
Your Complete Stress Proofing Programme, Leon Chaitow (Thorsons, 1984)
How to Meditate, Lawrence Le Shan (Turnstone, 1983)
Bach Flower Therapy, Mechthild Scheffer (Thorsons, 1986)

Professional Help

Osteopathy, Leon Chaitow (Thorsons, 1982)
Chiropractic: A Patient's Guide, (Thorsons, 1987)
Homoeopathy, Keith Scott and Linda A. McCourt (Thorsons, 1982)
The Healing Power of Acupuncture, Michael Nightingale (Javelin Books)
The Alternative Health Guide, Brian Inglis and Ruth West (Michael Joseph, 1983)

Useful Addresses

British Naturopathic and Osteopathic Association
Frazer House, 6 Netherhall Gardens, London NW3 5RR (01-435 8728)
(literature, speakers, and directory of registered practitioners)

The British Register of Naturopaths
17 Castlegate, Berwick-upon-Tweed TD15 1JS (0298 306477)

General Council and Register of Osteopaths
1-4 Suffolk Street, London SW1Y 4HG (01-839 2060) (literature and
directory)

The College of Osteopaths
110 Thornhill Road, Thames Ditton, Surrey KT7 0UW (01-398 3308)

British Chiropractic Association
5 First Avenue, Chelmsford, Essex CM1 1RX (0245 358487) (literature
and directory)

National Institute of Medical Herbalists
41 Hatherley Road, Winchester, Hampshire SO22 6RR (0962 68776)

British Acupuncture Association and Register
34 Alderney Street, London SW1V 4EU (01-834 1012/3353) (handbook,
directory, and speakers)

Traditional Acupuncture Society
11 Grange Park, Stratford-upon-Avon, Warwickshire CV37 6XH (0789
298798)

Register of Traditional Chinese Medicine
7a Thorndean Street, London SW18 4HE (01-947 1879)

International Register of Oriental Medicine
Green Hedges House, Green Hedges Avenue, East Grinstead, Sussex RH19 1DZ (0342 313106)

British Homoeopathic Association
27a Devonshire Street, London W1N 1RJ (01-935 2163) (literature and lists of medical homoeopaths)

Society of Homoeopaths
47 Canada Grove, Bognor Regis, West Sussex PO21 1DW (0243 860678) (qualified non-doctor homoeopaths)

British Hypnotherapy Association
67 Upper Berkeley Street, London W1 (01-723 4443)

National Federation of Spiritual Healers
Old Manor Farm Studio, Church Street, Sunbury-on-Thames, Middlesex TW16 6RG (0932 783164)

The Radionic Association
Baerlein House, Goose Green, Deddington, Oxford OX5 4SZ (0869 38852) (information and lists of practitioners)

International Institute of Reflexology
28 Hollyfield Avenue, London N11 3BY (01-368 0865)

British Wheel of Yoga
80 Leckhampton Road, Cheltenham, Gloucestershire GL53 0BN (0242 524889)

Yoga Biomedical Trust
P O Box 140, Cambridge CB1 1PU (0223 65771)

British T'ai Chi Chuan Association
7 Upper Wimpole Street, London W1M 7TD (01-935 8444)

Society of Teachers of the Alexander Technique
10 London House, 266 Fulham Road, London SW10 9EL (01-351 0828)

Action Against Allergy
43 The Downs, London SW20 8HG

National Society for Research into Allergy
P O Box 45, Hinckley, Leicester LE10 1JY (0455 635212)

The Soil Association
86 Colston Street, Bristol BS1 5BB (0272 290661) (The association has a continually up-dated list of approved organic food growers)

Dr Edward Bach Centre
Mount Vernon, Sotwell, Wallingford, Oxon OX10 0PZ (0491 39489) (The centre supplies remedies, books and advice on treatment with the Bach Flower Remedies)

The British Touch for Health Association
39 Browns Road, Surbiton, Surrey KT5 8ST (01-399-3215)

Products and Manufacturers

Food and nutrition

Soya milk.

is generally available in cartons — use the sugar-free type. Soya desserts also available in cartons in flavours such as vanilla, carob, strawberry. Recommended manufacturers — Plamil Foods Ltd., Granose Foods Ltd., Soya Health Foods Ltd., Provamel.

Margarine.

The most suitable brands are the sunflower oil, unhydrogenated, low-sodium margarine made by *Vitaquel* and *Vitasieg*. These are generally available from health food stores and high quality grocers.

Tahini.

Sesame seed paste for adding to fruit salads and for use in dressings is available from health food stores, ethnic stores, delicatessens, and some supermarkets. Recommended brands: *Cypressa*, *Harmony*.

Tofu.

Soya bean curd for use in various savouries and desserts as an alternative to milk and cheese. Available from health food stores and Chinese supermarkets.

Pure fruit jams.

These are suitable for hypoglycaemic subjects and diabetics. They are made only with the fruit and the fruit sugar content does not cause the same problems as sugar. Available from health food stores and supermarkets. Whole Earth products recommended.

Coffee substitutes. These are generally made from barley, figs, and chicory. The most palatable is *Pionier*, available from health food stores and imported from Switzerland by Inter-Medics Ltd.

Vitamin and mineral supplements. A wide choice of supplements are available from health food stores of varying quality and strength. Some are also available by mail order. Choose brands which are prepared using natural ingredients and with hypo-allergenic formulations. Recommended manufacturers — Healthcrafts Ltd., Nature's Own, Blackmores Laboratories Ltd., Lamberts Dietary Products Ltd., Larkhall Laboratories Ltd.

Celloid mineral supplements. By Blackmores Laboratories, available from practitioners only.

Tonics

A wide range of formulations of ginseng, pollen, royal jelly, vitamin E, propolis, and evening primrose oil, are available from health food stores. The following are just a few examples:

Ginseng plus pollen. Manufactured by Cernelle.
Polliforce. Manufactured by Cernelle; contains 18 amino acids and vitamin B6 with pollen.
Pollen-E-Vite. Manufactured by Healthcrafts.
Ginseng, Pollen, and Vitamin E. Manufactured by FSC Food Supply Co.
Regina Royal Jelly. Fresh royal jelly in a wheatgerm oil base with soya lecithin, manufactured by Wardglen.
Propolis pastilles with eucalyptus..

Herbal and homoeopathic

Dried herbs may be obtained from some health food stores and herbal suppliers. Many health food stores have herbal combinations available.

> *Sambucus complex*. Herbal and vitamin formulation by Blackmores Laboratories.
>
> *Dr Madaus Oligoplex preparations*. Imported by Inter-Medics Limited available from practitioners only.
>
> *New Era Combination H*. Together with other biochemic tissue salts this combination for hay fever is available from health food stores and certain chemists.
>
> *Homoeopathic medicines*. Some homoeopathic medicines available from health food stores and certain chemists. Most are made by Nelsons, Ainsworths, or Weleda. Mail service and personal callers can choose from wider range at Nelsons, 73 Duke Street, Grosvenor Square, London W1M 6BY (01-629 3118) and Ainsworth's, 38 New Cavendish Street, London W1 (01-935 5330).

Special equipment

Ionizers. Available from health food stores and medical supply shops. Leading manufacturers are Amcor (who also combine ionizers with air filters), Medion, and Mountain Breeze. Leaflets and price lists may be obtained from the manufacturers:

> Amcor (Appliances) Ltd., Amcor House, 19 Woodfield Road, Paddington, London W9 2BA (01-289 4433).
>
> Medion Ltd., Medion House, PO Box 557, New Milton, Hampshire BH25 5YF (0425) 638205).
>
> Mountain Breeze Air Ionizers, 6 Priorswood Place, East Pimbo, Skelmersdale, Lancashire WN8 9QB (0695 21155).

Hay Fever Helmet. Manufactured by R.H. Hinchliffe & Sons Ltd., 39 High Street, Pershore, Worcesterhire WR10 1EU (0386 555566), from whom information and prices may be obtained.

Index

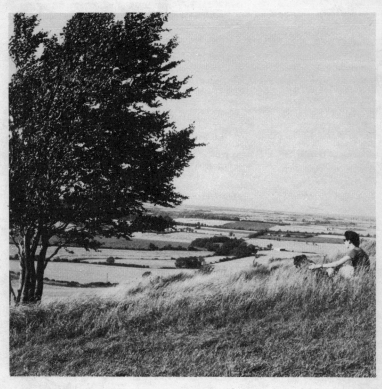

. . . pleasures regained.